SPICE DIET

SPICE UP SLIM DOWN

KALPNA WOOLF

C33444

D1147027

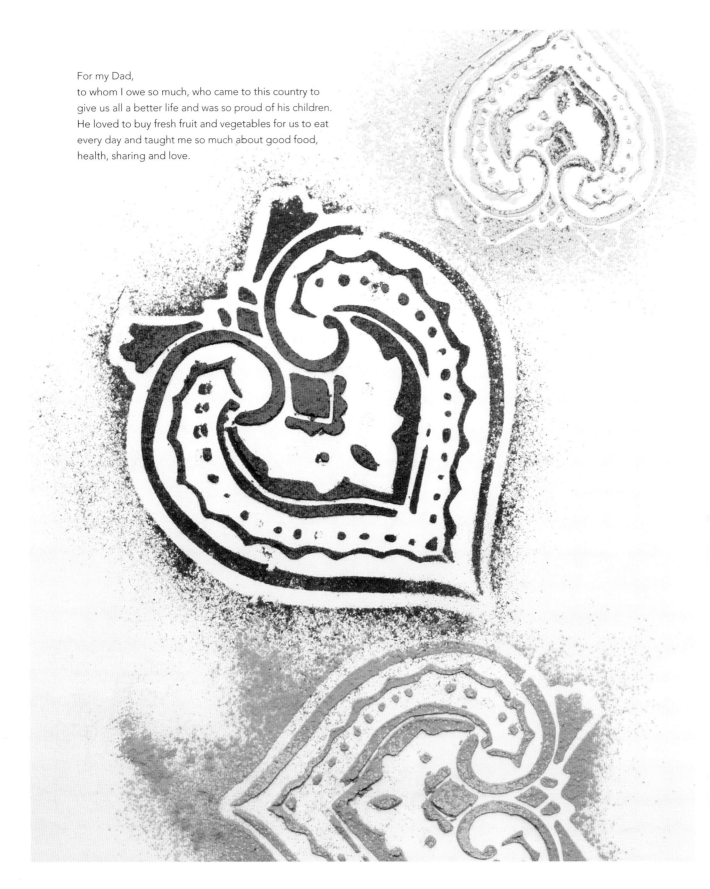

For my Dad,
to whom I owe so much, who came to this country to
give us all a better life and was so proud of his children.
He loved to buy fresh fruit and vegetables for us to eat
every day and taught me so much about good food,
health, sharing and love.

Contents

Introduction

Spices are powerhouses of flavour and health with the crucial benefit of being calorie and fat free. *Spice Diet* is a simple and healthy way to enjoy tasty food whilst also maintaining good health. This is not an invented contemporary fad; it has a strong foundation in centuries' old knowledge and traditions. *Spice Diet* reveals the secrets of one of the oldest and most valued, mystically powerful food sources known to mankind, and shows how spices can have a dramatic impact on our health, lifestyle and well-being.

Spice Diet guarantees weight loss whilst allowing you to enjoy flavourful food at every meal. Western tastes are ever more receptive to spices: from traditional (cloves, cinnamon, fennel); Indian (chilli, garam masala, turmeric, coriander) and Mexican (smoked chipotle chillies); to Chinese (Szechuan, Five spice, star anise) and Middle Eastern spices (Sumac, Za'atar, Ras el-Hanout). Yet we still know very little about their history and ability to improve our diets. This book unlocks their magic, fusing traditional spice secrets with simple, modern recipes.

I was brought up eating Indian spices and home-cooked food. However, when I moved away from home, I moved away from my 'food roots' too and was tempted by the growing proliferation of fast food. Instant food availability and the addictive effect of high fat, high salt, sugars and colours. I soon began to feel and look tired and began to put on weight. Even when I cut down on calories and felt I was eating less, I was still hungry and not managing my weight well.

Over the years I began to learn more about food and the effects of it on our health, energy levels and our weight. I realised that I wanted to eat healthily and feel full; to enjoy my food and to have a good relationship with it. But I didn't want to eat bland, flavourless and often insipid-looking 'diet' foods. I wanted to eat food with lots of flavour, to enjoy dishes from around the world, and share foods with my family. I discovered that when I balanced spices with healthy food my weight reduced and then stayed down.

Spice Diet is very much the story of the food journey I have travelled: from my roots growing up in a traditional Indian family in London; to university where, whilst studying Russian, I lived in Soviet Russia; returning home to learn how to cook traditional British dishes; and travelling since to experience cuisines first hand in Iran, China, Italy and then Thailand, Morocco, Mexico, the Mediterranean, the Far East and West Africa.

I still use spices every day – I love the tastes, flavours and the good feeling I get from just cooking a meal with them. Seeing the rich colour when I add turmeric to a dish, I am instantly transported to the bustling alleys of Old Delhi where turmeric powder is piled high in large sacks. Spices are sumptuous in colour, taste and history, evoking wonderful journeys across deserts, land and sea, to countries where they are so valuable they have been used as legal tender.

Spice are relished not only for their taste, but also because they come with stories of their health powers from one generation to another. My family and many Indian people I know, use remedies made from spices still for many ailments and strength. If anyone in my family has a bad tummy, everyone rushes for the carom seeds which are then mixed with a sprinkling of salt and swallowed down with a little warm water: a remedy going as far back as my great, great, grandmother.

As well as these family anecdotes, we now see scientific research confirming the health properties of spices. Turmeric has been used as an anti-inflammatory for years in Ayurvedic medicine and now scientific research shows that an active compound in turmeric, curcumin, could help reduce inflammation.

Cooking with spices really doesn't have to be intimidating or difficult. In *Spice Diet* I hope to demystify this and show how easily spices can be incorporated into our daily eating habits whilst capitalising on all those benefits to our health and well-being. That really is the magic allure of spices.

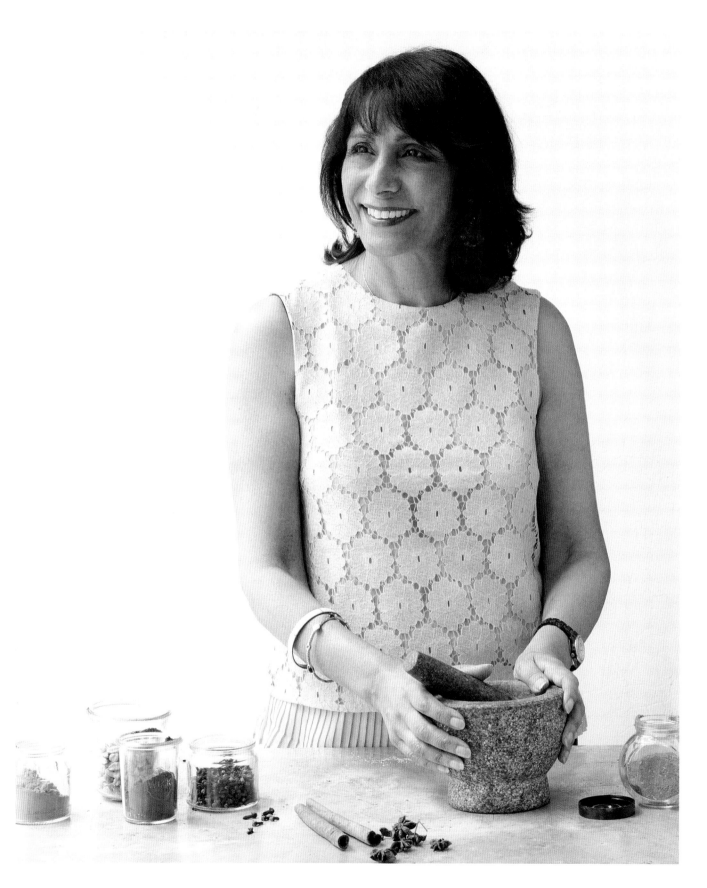

The Power of Spices

Spices are part of the world's food, trade and medicinal history. History recounts stories of colourful traders travelling from around the world on horseback, on ships and on foot handing over gold and silver coins for bags of wonderful spices. World markets teetered and thrived on the price of spices. Fantastic legends were weaved about the difficulty and rarity of spices so that the price could be held high (Arab traders told stories of cinnamon being carried by huge birds high into their nests. The birds would be lured down by tempting meats and, as they returned with the heavy meat, the nest would fall down with the cinnamon). Spices came from all over the world and, like plants, slowly germinated in parts of the world from which they hadn't originated.

When we think of spice traders, we think of men journeying from the East, but trade history shows a complex network from all over the world in the sale and use of spices – from India to Egypt to England to South America, China and to Africa and back again. Records go as far back as to at least the ancient Egyptians. For centuries spices have been traded for their taste, their healing powers and their preservative properties. This made them valuable and even gave some of them mystical powers; for example, cumin was thought to be 'strength-giving' so was carried by the Romans on their long marches and added to staple foods like bread. Some spices were used to ward off evil. Spices that 'warm' when eaten, like cinnamon, chilli and cardamom, were thought of as aphrodisiacs and were prescribed to 'warm up' lovemaking too! Early Chinese archives mention using spices with herbs to support overall health.

Before refrigeration, certain spices were discovered to be good preservatives for curing meats so they could be kept longer. This power raised their value enormously and, of course, the aroma of certain spices helped to overpower the sometimes pungent smell of the meat.

Records going back to Before Christ (BC) show that spices have been used for health and as medicines. Certain spices were burned as a remedy for headaches and others were used to work as

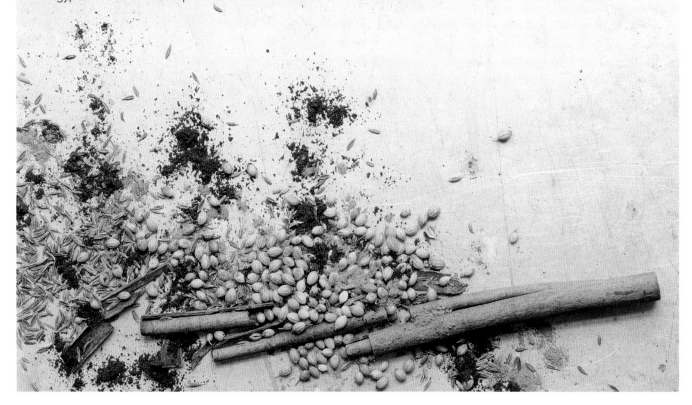

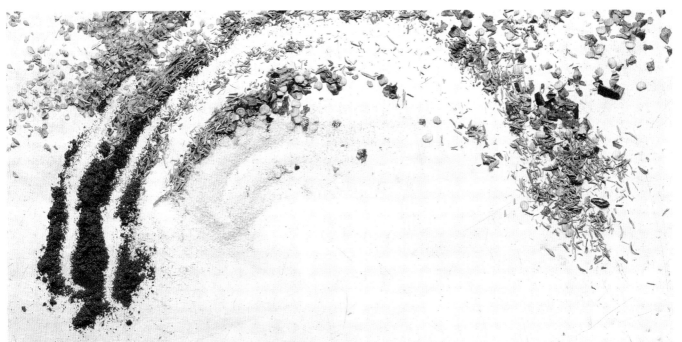

anaesthetics and to heal wounds more quickly. Coriander seeds have been found in Egyptian tombs and they have been cited in records as being used for headaches and muscular pain. What is interesting is that not all the spices recorded in Egyptian times were indigenous to Egypt, so they must have been carried from other parts of the world, and certainly cinnamon was one of those spices.

While spices were used for health, they were also used to flavour food and drink, including wine. Their exotic nature and their cost meant that wealthy people would use them as a way of showing off their prosperity and culinary skills.

Always Natural

Like many people, my personal food journey has led me to question where my food comes from. Making good food choices and making the right decisions about what I eat is very important to me. Time and again studies show that natural foods are better for your health. So many foods that we consume nowadays have been manufactured and tampered with, and this is particularly true of flavours. For years, artificial E numbers and flavour enhancers have been added to our foods to improve the taste, but their impact on our health hasn't always been positive. Even now, it is still sometimes hard to decipher what the ingredients are in many of the foods we buy.

Spices are powerful because they provide huge bursts of flavour and give great health benefits. All spices come from natural sources – seeds, barks, fruits, vegetables, etc. They have nothing added and no colours, sweeteners or preservatives. However, do read the ingredients on the packet in case salts or anything unnatural has been added to them.

Fear of Cooking with Spices

People often tell me that they are nervous about using spices because they don't understand the taste or the quantities to use. It's easy when you know the flavours of each spice and experimenting isn't a bad thing. All spices have a distinct flavour and it is about getting to know what each one tastes like. It's best to try the taste by cooking the spice rather than trying it in its natural form. Ground turmeric tastes bitter and earthy as a raw powder but delicious when cooked in rice or with vegetables or meat. Combining spices is also a good idea. Try using a single spice and then adding more. For example, a little chilli added to a dish will enhance the flavour, but as you add another spice, such as ground coriander, this will add another layer to the flavour to give a more complex taste. My spice rubs (see pp.16–19) are a good and easy way of learning how to combine spices.

How Does It Work?

Spice Diet is a healthy, flavourful way of eating based on centuries-old traditions of combining tasty spices with fresh ingredients to lose weight and maintain energy. It is a simple way of eating for the whole of your life. Most diets involve a 'crash and burn' timeframe but this is exactly why most diets tend not to work in the long term. For so long people have tried everything to lose weight or to maintain a good weight through short quick-fix diets, and while these diets may help to lose weight temporarily, statistics show that 95 per cent of dieters will fail to maintain weight loss. Diets tend to make you change your normal eating habits, deny yourself eating certain foods, and eat boring, bland foods you don't enjoy, or grapple with complicated meal plans. Often, you have to eat these dishes on your own while everyone around you is enjoying their meals. Dieting is thought of as a temporary fix with an end date. It is not seen as lifestyle change, so mentally most people are counting the days to when their diet is over. However, research also shows that if you can enjoy your meals, feel positive about the foods you are eating, because of their taste and nutrition, and share them with family and friends, you are more likely to succeed. *Spice Yourself Slim* is packed with recipes that you can enjoy and will help you to be successful in your diet.

Each recipe uses simple, natural ingredients and combines them with one or a combination of healthy spices to create wonderful low-fat dishes. For example, try rubbing a tablespoon of sumac (a wonderful Middle Eastern berry-coloured spice) into a few pieces of chicken then stir-frying them with a little olive oil, and you will have a delicious, zesty-flavoured chicken dish. The sumac doesn't add any calories at all. Alternatively, add cumin seeds to fresh vegetables before cooking and a sprinkling of roasted ground cumin at the end, and you will have a tantalising plate of food. You will also feel good as the cumin contains iron and other vitamins.

Spice Diet will show you which spices you need. I have used ten spices that are normally found in most kitchen storecupboards as well as some exciting new spices which I hope you will enjoy trying.

Using the Recipes

Breakfast and lunch recipes serve two people, but they will all work for four and there are tips on how to upscale the dishes. Dinner, entertainment and dessert dishes all serve four people. There are also many vegetarian dishes in the book and alternatives are given to satisfy the carnivores.

There are recipes for every day and also for light meat-free Mondays (see the meal planner on p.12). If you can't do this on a Monday, try to do one day a week based on this principle. Starting the week with a quieter eating day is an excellent way of cleansing the body. I believe that it also sharpens the mind. Having one day a week without meat will not only give your digestion a rest, but as you will eat more vegetables, herbs, beans, etc. you will have a day packed with more nutrients. It is also good for the environment, as considerably more greenhouse gases are produced in meat production, which has a detrimental effect on the environment.

Breakfast
Start the day well with energising, cleansing drinks and prepare your mind and body for the day ahead. A warm drink of ginger and fennel seeds or fresh mint is a great way of gently waking up your digestion and getting your body ready to receive a lovely, filling health-boosting breakfast. The breakfasts are designed to keep you feeling full, and to give you a healthy and energetic start to the day ahead. They will also keep your sugar levels stable, so you won't be tempted to reach for bad snacks.

In between meals, I recommend continuing to drink warm or cold spice-infused drinks, such as fennel tea, ginger and lemon drinks, and Golden Tea (see p.169). These drinks will keep you energised and keep your digestion and stomach soothed and happy until lunch.

Spicetastic lunches and effortless dinners
The lunch recipes range from warming soups with Moroccan spices, crunchy Asian salads and high-protein spicy fish or chicken dishes all filled with the flavour of spices, which will keep you revitalised through the afternoon.

Evenings are usually packed with things to do and we are often tired, but it's important to end the day with a good meal that doesn't take too long to prepare. Quick, easy, effortless dinners with lovely flavours are a key part of the *Spice Diet*. Being able to prepare a meal in the evening, which everyone wants to share, is a great way of unwinding and is a real de-stressor. Not worrying about what to cook is helped if you have spices in your cupboard and you know how to use them, as you can make any simple dish more exciting. Spice rubs are a great shortcut way of introducing a big shot of flavour to food quickly. It's also important not to eat too heavily at dinnertime so your digestion isn't continuing to work as you sleep – this won't help you sleep well. I suggest a warm herbal tea made with a digestive like fennel, peppermint and cardamom before you go to bed.

Tantalising sweet treats

There are days when we need something sweet to eat. *Spice Diet* offers some delicious treats for those days without devastating your calorie intake! These are healthy and gorgeous desserts with exotic spices like cardamom, saffron and vanilla, so you won't reach for the puddings with refined sugars and fats.

When you want to impress

Spice Diet is all about sharing food and not having to eat differently from your family and friends. In this book there are recipes that you can share but also show off when you have friends and family round. These entertainment recipes look beautiful and taste magnificent. They will look like you have spent a lot of time in the kitchen putting them together, but in fact they are very simple to do. You won't feel guilty eating these as they are low fat and are positively nutritious.

When you want an easy diet plan

Spice Diet gives you a 14-day meal plan so that you don't have to decide what you want to eat every day and you can rotate this for as long as you like. Full of tasty, nutritious foods and snacks, the Kick-starter Plan chapter (see p.10) will give you advice and a plan to follow to make life easy for yourself. Every recipe in this book has a calorie count attached to it.

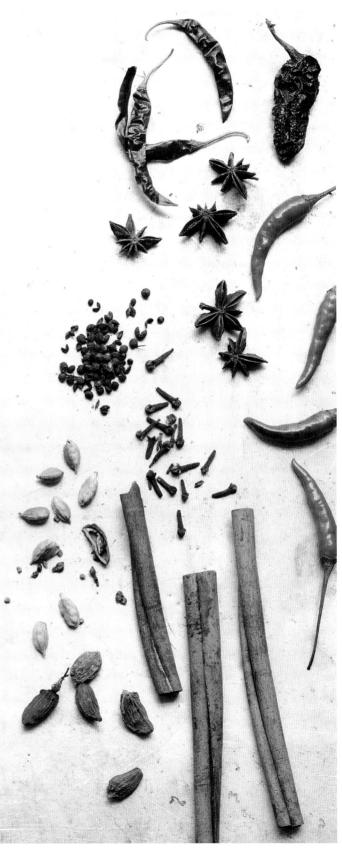

Kick-starter Plan

Sometimes we need a bit of help to kick-start a new way of eating or to help us plan our week's food better. This easy-to-follow meal plan will help you get ready for a new, long-lasting way of eating. It is not a quick fix, but a sensible, healthy way.

This plan includes all the foods we want to eat and dishes we can share, so no more depriving yourself or eating bland food, sitting in a corner on your own! Each dish contains good spices, which will taste lovely and also help to improve your health.

The meal plan includes delicious filling breakfasts that will keep you fuelled until lunchtime, but also a variety of healthy snacks if you do feel hungry. The weekends include indulgent but healthy breakfasts and dinners, which will make you feel in a holiday mood. These are also all good to share with family and friends.

You can mix and match the breakfasts, lunches and dinners and pick from any of the days except for Mondays. Mondays are designed to be light and meat free. This is a day of cleansing, but with plenty of good, flavourful food – you won't go hungry or have to eat dull, insipid meals.

Before you start, there are a few key things that will improve your diet and make you feel good.

Firstly, how you feel at the start of the day is often dictated not only by how you slept but also by when and what you have eaten the night before. If you sleep badly, your digestion will be out of sorts and your lack of energy will push you towards food cravings. In short, if you are tired your blood-sugar levels will fall, and as your energy levels tumble, this will cause cravings for sugary foods.

To prepare yourself for a good night's sleep, the basic simple rules are:

- Don't eat too late – eating drives your digestive system at a time when you want it to remain calm.
- Taking a warm bath with soothing ingredients will help you get a restful night.
- Sip a soothing drink of warm water with calming fennel seeds and fresh mint leaves 30 minutes before you go to sleep.
- Make the atmosphere in your room calm – no TV, phones or electronic gadgets, as these stimulate the brain at a time when we want the brain to rest.

In the morning, I recommend to start the day with a cleansing drink. Warm water with a healing spice, such as ginger, can help flush out any toxins in the body and get the digestion working. Ginger cleanses, detoxifies and as an anti-inflammatory it's great for joints, and works to fend off illnesses.

Fresh herbs and lemon mixed with spices work well in warm drinks and taste good too. I recommend drinking these throughout the day, alternating the spices for a different taste and also adding honey to help stop sweet cravings. Cinnamon is good in the afternoon when your sugar levels are flagging, while cloves support the immune system, and you can add honey or lemon to help with the taste. I have also included a variety of warm good-for-you drinks, for example, cayenne pepper added to warm water with a dash of lemon and ginger is good as a metabolism booster. The supreme champion of healthy drinks is Golden Tea or Golden Milk (p.163). This is a hot drink packed with anti-inflammatory and antiseptic turmeric and fresh ginger made tasty with milk, honey and ginger.

Some common-sense rules are:
- Shop for the ingredients ahead of time.
- Always start the day with a warm, cleansing drink.
- Never skip breakfast.
- Snacks are optional – eat these only if hungry.
- Eat dinner as early as you can and at least 3 hours before you go to bed.
- Drink a warm, cleansing drink (fennel and mint) before you go to bed.
- Watch your portion sizes.
- Try to walk every day – you don't have to go to the gym or an exercise class several times a week, but walking briskly every day for around 20 minutes will keep you healthy.

Shopping List

Opposite is a list of spices and flavours to add to your shopping list. There is a list of 'storecupboard spices' for any dried ingredients you can keep for longer than fresh and a list of 'fresh flavours' that will need to bought more frequently and replenished. I have compiled this list using the regularly used herbs and flavours from the Kick-starter Plan (p.12–15) and the dried spices from the six basic spice rub recipes (p.18–19). This list is by no means exhaustive, nor is every item essential for introducing spice to your diet; it's there to help you get started and to pick and choose recipes that suit your tast and lifestyle. Please note that although the dried spices can be stored in the cupboard, they don't last forever (see p.19).

Storecupboard spices:
- Bay leaves (dried and fresh)
- Black peppercorns
- Cardamom pods (black and green)
- Carom seeds
- Cayenne Pepper
- Chilli flakes
- Chilli powder
- Chipotle Chillies
- Cinnamon (ground)
- Cinnamon sticks
- Cloves
- Coriander seeds
- Cumin seeds
- Fennel seeds
- Fenugreek seeds
- Garlic powder (dried)
- Kashmiri chillies
- Mexican Oregano (dried)
- Mint (dried)
- Mustard seeds
- Oregano (dried)
- Paprika
- Thyme (dried)
- Turmeric (ground)
- Star Anise
- Sumac
- Szechuan peppers
- Za'atar

Fresh flavours:
- Basil
- Coriander
- Curry leaves (fresh)
- Galangal
- Garlic
- Ginger
- Lemongrass
- Lemons
- Limes
- Mint
- Parsley
- Red chillies
- Thyme/lemon thyme
- Turmeric root

Week 1

DAY	DRINK	BREAKFAST	SNACK
MONDAY (light/meat-free day	Warm water with fennel and ginger	Get-Up-and-Go Breakfast Smoothie (p.29) 62 KCAL	Handful of nuts and seeds. Chew fennel seeds. Drink warm water with honey and fennel 157 KCAL
TUESDAY	Warm water with turmeric, ginger, lemon and honey	Superfood Quinoa Porridge with Apple and Cinnamon (p.27) 291 KCAL	Handful of nuts and seeds and chew fennel seeds. Drink Warm water with fennel 134 KCAL
WEDNESDAY	Warm water with cardamom seeds and mint	Labneh Sumac and Fig Breakfast (p.34) 361 KCAL	2 tbsp Beetroot and Cumin Dip (p.142) with carrot sticks. Drink warm water with fennel and mint 46 KCAL
THURSDAY	Warm water with lemongrass, ginger and basil	Cardamom-Infused Porridge (p.26) 203 KCAL	1 piece Ginger and Cardamom Snack Jack (p.144). Drink warm water with fennel and mint 78 KCAL
FRIDAY	Warm water with cayenne pepper, ginger and lemon	Mixed Berry Compote with Cardamom and Cinamon Porridge (p.26) 241 KCAL	2 tbsp Beetroot and Cumin Dip (p.142) with carrot sticks 46 KCAL
SATURDAY	Warm water with turmeric, lemon and ginger or Golden Tea (p.169)	Spectacular Fennel and Orange-Drenched Smoked Salmon (p.24) 143 KCAL	Handful of nuts and seeds. Chew fennel seeds. Drink warm water with honey and fennel 157 KCAL
SUNDAY	Warm water with star anise and clove	Middle Eastern Spinach and Egg Stack (p.32) 139 KCAL	1 apple 51 KCAL

Nuts = Brazil, almonds or walnuts

LUNCH	SNACK	DINNER	TOTAL CALORIES
Immunising Turmeric Soup (p.51) and 2 oatcakes or 2 rice cakes 267 KCAL	1 sliced apple topped with 2 tbsp plain yogurt sprinkled with ground cinnamon 97 KCAL	Mediterranean Sumac Roast Vegetables with Butter Beans (p.93) 239 KCAL	822 KCAL
Caramelised Pumpkin, Goat's Cheese and Winter Fruit Salad (p.40) 341 KCAL	4–5 dried apricots, small handful of seeds 91 KCAL	Two-Spice Salmon with Magnificent Mango Salsa (p.81) 397 KCAL	1254 KCAL
Super Crunchy Asian Salad (p.66) 214 KCAL	Fresh berries (around 30g/1oz) and plain yogurt with ground cinnamon 53 KCAL	Mum's Curcumin Loaded Daal (p.99) with Cauliflower Rice (p.98) or wholemeal pitta bread 418 KCAL	1092 KCAL
Immunising Turmeric Soup (p.51) and 2 oatcakes or 2 rice cakes 267 KCAL	½ papaya drizzled with fresh lime and black pepper 73 KCAL	Thai-Spiced Seared Tuna with Fennel and Blood Orange Salad (p.110) 367 KCAL	988 KCAL
Indian Reviving Tomato Shorba (p.54) 150 KCAL	1 piece Ginger and Cardamom Snack Jack (p.144) 69 KCAL	Singapore Satay Sticks with Mooli Slaw (p.94) 243 KCAL	749 KCAL
South Indian Hot and Sour Soup (p.68) with 2 rice cakes 288 KCAL	1 apple with a small handful of seeds 85 KCAL	Saigon-Style Fillet Beef (p.129) 267 KCAL	940 KCAL
Hot and Fragrant Tom Yam Soup (p.52) 58 KCAL	½ papaya drizzled with fresh lime and black pepper 73 KCAL	Uplifting Lemon Coriander Chicken with Roast Peppers (p.107) 332 KCAL	653 KCAL

Week 2

DAY	DRINK	BREAKFAST	*SNACK*
MONDAY (light/meat-free day)	Warm water with ginger and lemon	Watermelon Cinnamon and Cottage Cheese Bowl (p.30) 248 KCAL	Handful of nuts and seeds. Drink warm water with lemon, fennel and honey 157 KCAL
TUESDAY	Warm water with turmeric, ginger, lemon and honey	Star Anise and Cinnamon Porridge (p.26) 203 KCAL	2 tbsp Beetroot and Cumin Dip (p.142) with celery. Drink warm water with fennel and mint 77 KCAL
WEDNESDAY	Warm water with cayenne pepper, ginger and lemon	Superfood Quinoa Porridge with Apple and Cinnamon (p.27) 291 KCAL	1 piece Cardamom and Ginger Snack Jack (p.144) 78 KCAL
THURSDAY	Warm water with cardamom and cloves	Super-Boosted Turmeric and Black Pepper Smoothie (p.29) 394 KCAL	1 piece Ginger and Cardamom Snack Jack (p.144). Drink warm water with fennel and mint 78 KCAL
FRIDAY	Warm water with lemongrass, ginger and basil	Apple and Cinnamon Porridge (p.26) 216 KCAL	2 tbsp Beetroot and Cumin Dip (p.142) with carrot sticks. Drink warm water with fennel and ginger 77 KCAL
SATURDAY	Warm water with star anise and clove	Fennel and Orange-Drenched Smoked Salmon (p.24) 143 KCAL	Handful of nuts and seeds. Chew fennel seeds. Drink warm water with fresh mint and fennel 157 KCAL
SUNDAY	Warm water with fennel and mint or Golden Tea (p.163)	Middle Eastern Spinach and Egg Stack (p.32) 139 KCAL	Handful of seeds and apricots. Drink warm water with ginger and mint 91 KCAL

Nuts = Brazil, almonds or walnuts

LUNCH	SNACK	DINNER	TOTAL CALORIES
Super-Crunchy Asian Salad (p.66) 214 KCAL	1 apple with 2 tbsp plain yogurt and a sprinkle of ground cinnamon 91 KCAL	Sustaining Mexican Black Beans and Peppers (p.92) 214 KCAL	924 KCAL
Fresh Herb Maroque Tabbouleh with Minted Halloumi (p.46) 363 KCAL	1 kiwi fruit with plain yogurt and ground cinnamon 75 KCAL	Sumac-Dusted Hake with Super-Boosted Carom Seeds and Kale (p.104) 227 KCAL	945 KCAL
Mexicana Bean Tacos (p.60) 328 KCAL	½ papaya with lime and black pepper 73 KCAL	Szechuan-Style Chicken and Green Beans (p.113) 256 KCAL	1026 KCAL
Moroccan Chorba with Orzo (p.69) 140 KCAL	2 satsumas and some seeds 91 KCAL	Filling Freekeh Pilaf and Sumac Ricotta (p.80) 200 KCAL	903 KCAL
Vietnamese Chicken and White Cabbage Salad (p.44) 236 KCAL	1 piece Ginger and Cardamom Snack Jack (p.144) 78 KCAL	Quick Treat Mexican Red Rice (p.90) and Shaved Fennel Salad (p.138) 311 KCAL	918 KCAL
Indian Reviving Tomato Shorba (p.54) 150 KCAL	1 apple with 2 tbsp plain yogurt and cinnamon 97 KCAL	Thai-Spiced Tuna Steak with Fennel and Blood Orange Salad (p.110) 367 KCAL	914 KCAL
Healthy Sweet Potato and Spinach Cakes with Yogurt Raita (p.56) 255 KCAL	Mixed berries and seeds 48 KCAL	Roman Holiday Seafood Parcels (p.82) 225 KCAL	758 KCAL

Spice Rubs

A spice rub is just a combination of spices that give a distinct flavour. Spice rubs have been around for a long time – the well-known Chinese five spice is a combination of five spices, but sometimes more. The Moroccan ras el hanout is a spice mix of anything from at least 12 spices to many more and, of course, there is the ubiquitous curry powder, which is a mix of Indian spices, and garam masala found in most homes in North India.

These spice rubs serve as a ready-made, homemade combination of spices to enhance dishes, give nutritional benefits and a feast for the eyes – try rubbing the South Indian Spice Rub (p.18) onto a humble fish fillet and the result is an appealing, mouthwatering and nourishing meal. Or, make a zesty gremolata of fresh garlic, red chilli, fresh coriander, lemon zest and ground coriander then marinate tiger prawns or a salmon steak in this, and you will be licking your lips! All these dishes do not contain any extra calories – they are free and healthy.

Spice rubs are flavourful

There are certain 'flavours' that can be achieved by combining spices in a ready-made dry mix rather than mixing individual spices in the pan. Spice rubs take just minutes to make and are a quick, easy, convenient and exciting way of using spices and achieving a certain 'style' of food. So, if you want a tandoori-style meal, reach for the spice rub rather than a number of jars, sprinkle it on your fish or meat, and your food will come alive with a delicious tandoori taste.

Spice rubs make life easy

When you're busy and stressed out, brush a spice rub over some meat or fish or sprinkle over vegetables and transform a simple ingredient into a delicious meal. They are an ingenious way of making life easier and taking the headache out of deciding which spice to use or using loads of jars from the cupboard. Alternatively, you can transport yourself to the warm Mediterranean, the sultry medinas of Morocco and to Mexican pueblos and lift your mood. It only takes minutes to make up a batch and then you can create delicious, healthy spicy dishes in minutes.

Spice rubs are natural fast food

This is fast food, but made by you at home, so you're in control of the ingredients. This is the spice world equivalent of a ready meal. Spice-ready – to go! However, these rubs are not like the ready meals you buy. When making your spice rub, you will know exactly what goes into it. Your spice rub is always going to be nutritious, natural, delicious, flavourful, and with no unnatural colours, preservatives, sugars, sweeteners and other hidden ingredients.

Spice rubs are de-stressers

Cooking every day requires planning and often worrying about what to make and making sure you have shopped for all the ingredients. We don't always have space, time or the inclination to do this, so it is easy to reach for a ready meal or a takeaway, which will not always leave you feeling healthy or good. However, having a spice rub ready to cook with will relieve the tension and stress of deciding what to eat. Making a few of them will instantly give you a variety of meals you can cook and enjoy. As they say, variety is the spice of life! Research shows that eating when you are at ease and relaxed is very important in how well the nutrients are absorbed into your body to give you the full goodness from the food you are eating.

Spice rubs and learning about them are fun

Combining spices is a fun and easy way of using them. Why not prepare your spice rub with your children, as it helps them to understand spices and natural food and they will lose the fear of using spices from a young age?

Recipes Using the Spice Rubs

You can use these spice rubs in many different recipes and it will be quite fun to experiment. They all work well with meats, vegetables and fish.

Mediterranean

My Super-Herby Feel-Good Frittata (p.62)
Mediterranean Stuffed Aubergines (p.88)
Mediterranean Sumac Roast Vegetables
    with Butter Beans (p.93)
Roman Holiday Seafood Parcels (p.82)

Moroccan-Style

Moroccan Cinnamon and Preserved Lemon
    Chicken (p.125)
Speedy Aromatic Moroccan Chorba with Orzo (p.69)
Fresh Herb Maroque Tabbouleh with
    Minted Halloumi (p.46)
Tangiers Festive Fish (p.132)

Szechuan-Style

Flash-Fried Beef and Citrus Courgettini (p.72)
Szechuan-Style Chicken and Green Beans (p.113)
Chinese Pork Tenderloin with Braised Pak Choi
    and Baby Leeks (p.124)
Super-Crunchy Asian Salad (p.66)

Mexican

Mexicana Bean Tacos (p.60)
Fajita-Style Chicken (p.50)
Sustaining Mexican Black Beans and Peppers (p.92)
Steaming Mexican Seasoned Mussels (p.130)

Tandoori

An Indian Abroad Sunday Roast (p.118)
Easy and Lite Saucy Tandoori Chicken (p.84)
Chilli Tofu Kebabs with Beetroot and
    Onion Slaw (p.45)
Super-Quick Chargrilled Tandoori Tilapia (p.105)

South Indian

Spicy Veggie Kedgeree (p.36)
South Indian Hot and Sour Lentil Soup (p.68)
Keralan Masala Fish (p.58)
Comforting South Indian Rainbow Vegetables (p.78)

How to Make a Spice Rub

You need only three pieces of equipment:
- measuring spoons
- electric grinder (or pestle and mortar)
- a glass jar with tight-fitting lid

I generally use whole spices, which I roast and then grind, but you can use already ground spices and just combine them. Roasting gives spices a deeper flavour and doesn't take long to do. Just warm a heavy-based frying pan before adding the spices, then add them to the pan and gently roast them for a few minutes. Roasting releases the spice's oils and aroma as well as adding an intensity of flavour to the dish.

Whole spices versus powdered

Roasting whole spices introduces another level of aroma and taste to a dish. However, without an electric grinder it is difficult to pound some spices with a pestle and mortar, but it can be done and is certainly worth the effort. If you don't have an electric grinder, you can use ready-ground spices instead. My advice would be to buy the very best spices (organic if possible) and then combine them into a spice rub. A whole cinnamon stick can be added to Chinese and Indian spice rubs.

Dry/wet spice rubs

All the spice rubs can be turned into 'wet rubs' by adding a wet ingredient, such as yogurt, lemon, stock or oil.

Homemade Spice Rubs

Basic Spice Rub

Roast the whole spices together in a pan for 3–5 minutes, until the aromas are released. Grind your roasted spices into a fine powder and mix in the pre-ground spices. Store in an airtight jar.

Tandoori

Tandoori recipes originate from North India, where soft breads and pieces of meat and fish are marinatedin mouthwatering spices, threaded onto long skewers, and plunged into the charcoal heat of the tandoor. This is a fragrant and medium-hot mix of Indian spices, with an authenticity that is not always easy to find. The Kashmiri chillies give the spice rub a deep colour.

To make 25g/1oz/4 tbsp

8 cloves
5 medium Kashmiri chillies
6 tbsp coriander seeds
8 whole black cardamom pods
4 x 5cm/2in cinnamon sticks
2 tbsp ground turmeric
1tbsp chilli powder

Follow the instructions for the Basic Spice Rub.

South Indian

The heat of South India is often matched in food with hot chillies and flavours. This spice rub will transport you to the south of India, which is a fantastic mixture of cities full of beautiful ornate temples, the quiet lakes of Kerala and the tropical beaches of Goa. This spice mix is a heady combination of cassia bark, cumin seeds, coriander seeds, mustard seeds, fenugreek seeds, Kashmiri chillies, whole cardamom and turmeric.

To make 25g/1oz/4 tbsp

8 x 2.5cm/1in pieces cinnamon bark
2 tbsp cumin seeds
2 tbsp coriander seeds
1 tbsp mustard seeds
1 tsp fenugreek seeds
5 Kashmiri chillies
3 whole black cardamom pods
2 tbsp ground turmeric
2 tbsp chilli powder

Follow the instructions for the Basic Spice Rub, reserving the cardamom pods until after your roasted spices have been mixed with the pre-ground spices. Smash the cardamoms 2–3 times with a rolling pin and add to the mix.

Mexican

Chocolate and chilli sauces, ripe avocados, crisp corn kernels, black beans and smoky chillies – just a few of the foods we love from this cuisine, influenced by Aztecs, Spaniards, Texans and Mayan Indians. Mexican oregano has a more intense flavour than Mediterranean oregano, but if you can't get hold of it, use Mediteranrean.

To make 25g/1oz/4 tbsp

4 chipotle chillies (use 1 tbsp chilli flakes if you can't get chipotles)
4 tbsp coriander seeds
4 tbsp cumin seeds
2 tbsp paprika
2 tbsp Mexican dried oregano

Follow the instructions for the Basic Spice Rub.

Moroccan-Style

This mix reminds me of the tastes and smells of Morocco and the beautiful countries of North Africa. These are the wonderful spices of which you catch wafts when you walk through the labyrinthine streets of the medinas.

To make 30g/1oz/4 tbsp

3 tbsp cumin seeds
2 tbsp coriander seeds
1 tbsp paprika
1 tbsp ground turmeric
1 whole cinnamon stick

Follow the instructions for the Basic Spice Rub, reserving the cinnamon stick and adding to the jar at the end.

Mediterranean

This spice rub includes herbs that instantly evoke memories of the Mediterranean region. I went through a fanatical 'Italy' period – not wanting to travel anywhere else in the world – obsessed by its food and culture. This rub is inspired by my sunny, food-fuelled days in different parts of Italy. It is more of an aromatic spice rub with a nod to a slight chilli warmth. Based on the healthy diet of the Mediterranean – good and light – this is a mixture of herbs that are native to that region.

To make 25g/1oz/4 tbsp

4 tbsp dried oregano
4 tbsp dried thyme
2 tsp red mild chilli flakes
1 tsp paprika
1 tsp dried garlic powder
½ tsp fine sea salt

Simply measure the ingredients, mix together in a jar, seal with a lid and shake well. Store in an airtight jar away from sunlight.

Szechuan-Style

I wanted to create a spice rub that had a Chinese flavour but was indulgent, unique and included the distinctive taste of Szechuan pepper. This rub has quite an intense taste so use sparingly. Szechuan peppers remind me of ceremonial Chinese royal courts and heavy dragon-brocaded silk tapestries. Reminiscent of the Chinese five-spice mix, this spice rub has been up-scaled to include a truly magnificent spice – Szechuan pepper.

To make 25g/1oz/4 tbsp

2 tbsp Szechuan peppers
3 star anise
2 tbsp fennel seeds
5 cloves
½ tbsp black peppercorns
2.5cm/1in cinnamon stick
½ tsp salt

Follow the instructions for the Basic Spice Rub, or, place the whole spices on a baking tray and roast for 4–5 minutes in a warm oven until you can smell the Szechuan pepper, then remove immediately. Grind everything together to a fine powder. If there any husks left from the Szechuan peppers, sieve the powder. Mix in the salt and store in an airtight jar.

How to Store Spice Rubs

Spice rubs are just like individual spices. Keep them away from heat and moisture and store in airtight jars. Always label them so you know what they are and when you mixed them. They will last happily for 6–9 months, but after that they will lose their taste and colour. An indication that the rub is not doing well is if the colour is fading and becoming dull.

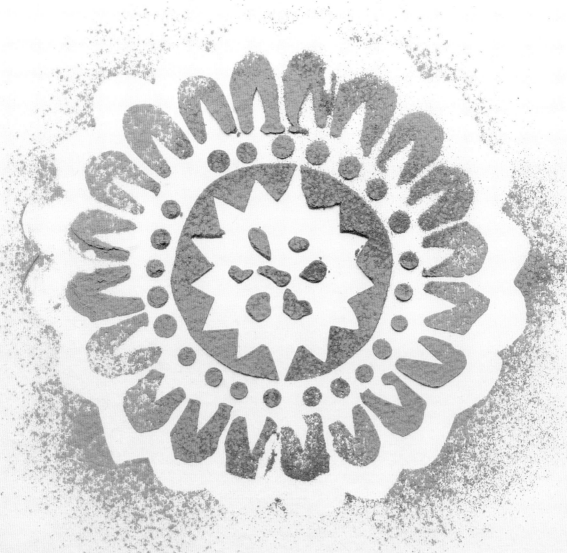

Start the Day: Breakfasts

After a night's sleep, your body needs a good breakfast, which will nurture it. It's been said many times before that breakfast is the most important meal of the day and too many of us either skip it altogether in the morning rush or don't eat well and properly. If you get this right, you set yourself up for the day ahead with plenty of energy and fuel that will not only keep you going, but stop you giving in to unhealthy snacks or eating more than you need at lunch.

With the simple addition of spices, such as cardamom, ginger and cinnamon, you can reinvent breakfast staples like porridge and eggs. Why not try something less familiar for breakfast, such as watermelon, figs, smoked salmon or kedgeree and create some tasty and energy-giving drinks or smoothies to set you up for the day?

211 KCAL

Aanda Bhourgee (Eggs Indian Style)

Serves 4

Ingredients

2 tbsp olive oil

2 garlic cloves, peeled and finely chopped

4 large spring onions (scallions), including green part, roughly chopped

½ tsp salt, or to taste

½ tsp ground turmeric

½ tsp ground coriander

1 medium chilli, finely chopped

2 large beef tomatoes (or equivalent amount in salad tomatoes), roughly chopped into cubes

a large handful of fresh coriander (cilantro), stems and leaves chopped separately

8 organic eggs

This is the dish that reminds me instantly of Sunday family breakfasts. When I visit my sister, everyone expects me to make a yummy wholesome breakfast. On a lazy Sunday morning, the delicious smell brings all the family out of bed, running down the stairs and sitting ready at the table. It's a great sharing dish, which will satisfy the whole family and keep them full and feeling good until lunchtime. Garlic, chilli, ground coriander and turmeric all combine in this dish to keep you healthy and strong.

Method

Heat the oil in a large frying pan over a low heat. Add the garlic and spring onion and sauté gently for 3–4 minutes until soft. Add the salt, turmeric, ground coriander and chilli, and cook gently for a couple of minutes. Mix in the tomatoes and coriander stems and cook for a further 2–3 minutes until the tomatoes are soft but not too mushy.

Break the eggs into a bowl and whisk lightly with a fork. Pour into the tomatoes and cook for 3–4 minutes, or until set. Check the seasoning, sprinkle over the coriander leaves and serve immediately.

Tip

This is excellent for a brunch or lunch too. Serve with hot toasted wholemeal pitta bread or a slice of rye or gluten-free bread. Increase the number of eggs from six to eight if having this for brunch or lunch and increase the cooking time of the eggs to 4–5 minutes, or until cooked to your liking.

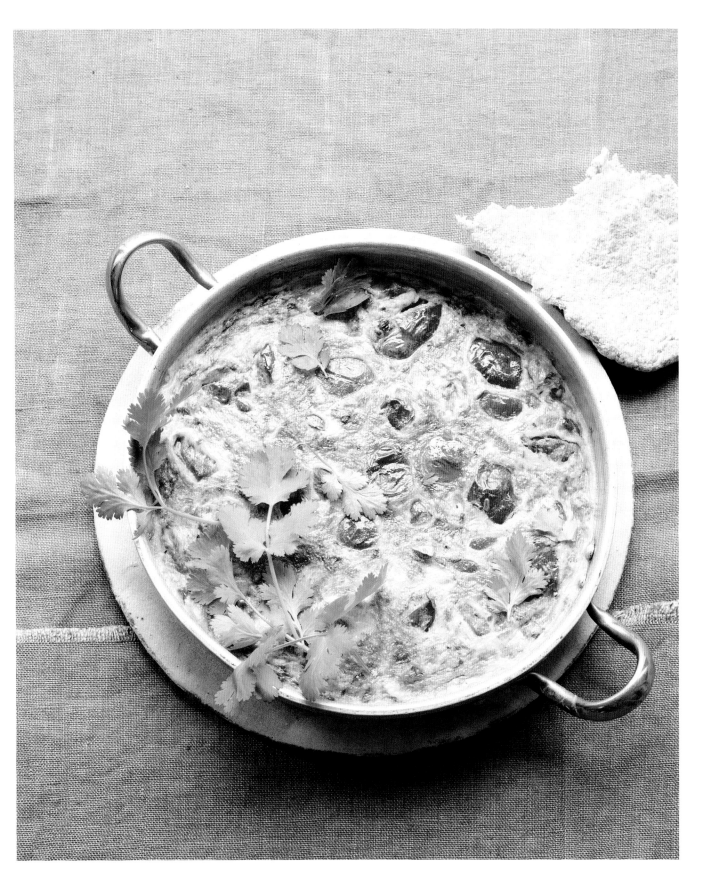

143 KCAL

Spectacular Fennel and Orange-Drenched Smoked Salmon

Serves 2

Ingredients

1 small bag (100g/3½oz) spinach
  leaves, washed
½ fennel bulb, thinly sliced
100g/3½oz smoked salmon

For the dressing

2 oranges, 1 juiced and ¼ zest
  finely grated and 1 peeled
  and sliced or segmented
¼ red chilli, deseeded and
  finely sliced
2 tsp finely chopped or grated
  fresh ginger
freshly ground black pepper
½ tsp balsamic vinegar
½ tsp olive oil
1 tsp Dijon mustard

I love to have a variety at breakfast and this breakfast instantly puts a smile on my face! During my kosher family days I ate a lot of smoked salmon and often combined it with chilli, lemon and black pepper to cut through the oiliness and to give it a kick. This is a breakfast that you will look forward to because it is a beautiful colour and is full of essential omega-3 fatty acids and vitamin C. The green salad leaves together with the fresh ginger will cleanse your stomach and have a calming effect, and the chilli will get your metabolism moving. This recipe is quick and easy as you can make the dressing ahead of time and keep it in the refrigerator for when you feel like making this salad.

Method

Mix all the dressing ingredients together in a jar and give it a good shake. Chill in the refrigerator. This can be made the night before and will keep for a few days.

Arrange the spinach leaves and fennel slices on a serving plate. Layer the smoked salmon slices over the top, then arrange the orange slices around the plate. Shake the dressing and sprinkle over the top of the salad. Serve.

Tips

- This is a good salad for lunch too and goes well with rye bread, black bread or a soft-boiled egg.
- The dressing is also delicious in many salads (e.g. chicken and avocado) so make some extra and keep it for use later.

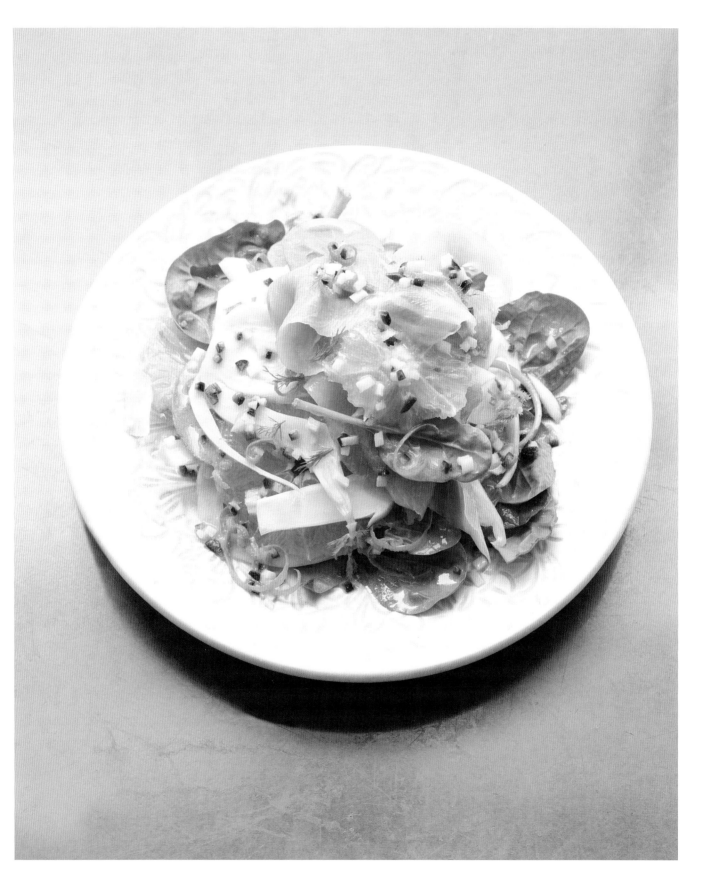

203 KCAL

Spice Up Your Porridge

Serves 2

Ingredients

80g/3¼oz/1 cup rolled oats
  (you can soak these overnight)
300ml/10½fl oz/1¼ cups milk or
  half milk/half water
a pinch of salt

Numerous studies have shown that starting your day with porridge is so good for you. Oats mixed with any milk (this can be lactose-free) provides a perfect meal packing a big punch of nutrients and lots of fibre. Fibre not only keeps you feeling full and gives you lasting energy, but also helps keep blood sugar levels on an even keel for the day. Adding spices will upscale the health benefits and punch even more in terms of nutrients and flavour. Here is a standard recipe for porridge and a few suggestions to spice it up.

Method

Place the oats and milk in a heavy-based saucepan and bring slowly to a simmer. Keep stirring all the time for 5–8 minutes. If the consistency is getting too thick, add a little more milk or water. Add the salt in the last minute of cooking.

Tip

Buy good-quality oats. The more they have been rolled, the faster they will cook and will be easier to digest. If you wish, you can soak the oats overnight as this can give the porridge a creamier taste and will be quicker to cook in the morning. To soak the oats, just put the oats and milk (or water) together in a bowl, cover and leave in the refrigerator. Almond, coconut or cow's milk are all good choices, or use half milk and half water, but the original Scottish recipe is made with only water. Remember to reduce the cooking time in the morning.

Spice Up Your Porridge Ideas
- Add 2 cardamom pods (smash lightly to bruise so that this infuses the milk) to the milk while warming the milk and top with a drizzle of honey.
- Poach a few cubes of rhubarb with grated fresh ginger, water and ½ teaspoon honey. Top your porridge with a spoonful of the rhubarb.
- Add in a star anise and cinnamon stick when soaking the oats overnight or when cooking the porridge.
- Mixed berry compote with cinnamon and cardamom: Put 50g/1¾oz/ ⅓ cup mixed fresh berries in a pan with 50ml/2fl oz/scant ¼ cup water. Add ½ cinnamon stick and warm through. Sprinkle ¼ teaspoon ground cardamom powder or a drizzle of honey over the top.
- Apple and walnut with grated nutmeg.
- Add cloves and a cinnamon stick to the milk and top with sliced apple.
- For a luxurious porridge, infuse the milk with a vanilla pod and top the porridge with black cherries or blueberries.
- Banana and cinnamon: Peel and slice a banana. Arrange on a grill pan and sprinkle over 1 teaspoon ground cinnamon. Place under a hot grill and, when browned, add to your porridge.

Superfood Quinoa Porridge with Apple and Cinnamon

Quinoa is packed with protein, is gluten free and has a low glycaemic index (GI) which means that it is absorbed more slowly into the bloodstream and will keep your blood sugar levels more stable. It will also keep you fuller for longer. Quinoa is a good alternative to oat porridge. Cinnamon gives this breakfast a natural sweetness. Cinnamon has many health properties: it's high in antioxidants, is an antiseptic and keeps your digestion working well.

Method

Pour the cold milk into a pan, mix in the quinoa and add the cinnamon stick. Bring to the boil then reduce the heat to a simmer, cover with a lid and leave to cook for 10 minutes.

Mix the grated apples and vanilla extract into the quinoa and cook for a further 2–3 minutes until thick and creamy. Remove the cinnamon stick, sprinkle the ground cinnamon over the top and the Brazil nuts (and the berries, if using). Eat hot.

Tip

Use coconut or almond milk if you prefer not to have lactose or want to go dairy free.

Serves 2

Ingredients

250ml/9fl oz/generous 1 cup low-fat milk, coconut milk or almond milk

100g/3½oz/½ cup quinoa

1 cinnamon stick

1 eating apple, cored and grated

¼ tsp vanilla extract

1 tsp ground cinnamon

2 tbsp chopped Brazil nuts

a few raspberries or blueberries (optional)

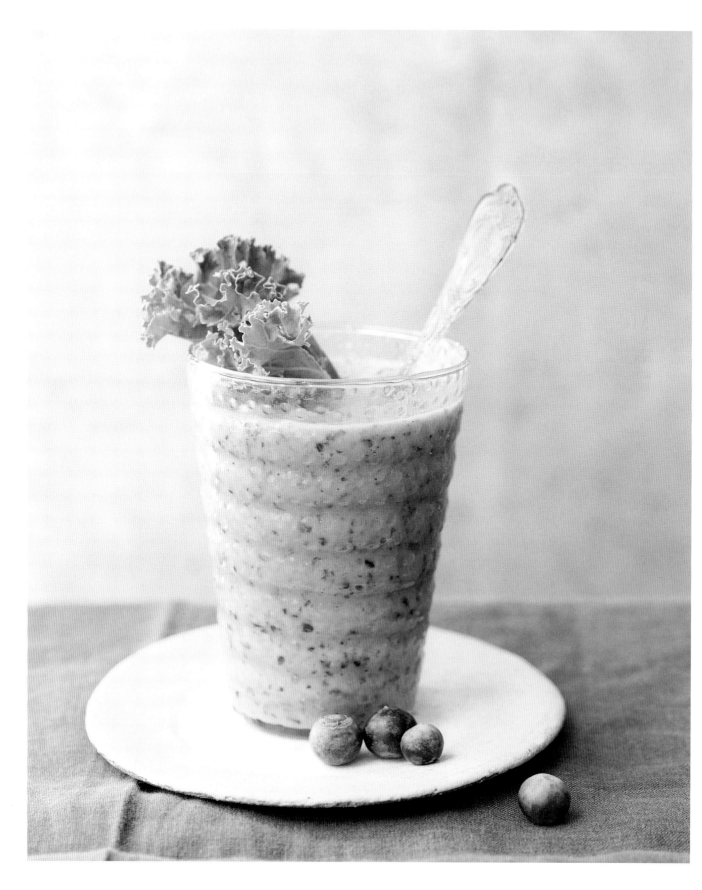

Get-Up-and-Go Smoothie

62 KCAL

Smoothies are a great way of packing antioxidants, vitamins and protein all in one glass and there are unlimited combinations that you can come up with. Adding spices, such as turmeric, ginger and chilli (optional), make the smoothies work even harder. Turmeric is a super-spice – anti-inflammatory, antiseptic and an all round spice to keep you well. Ginger will help the complex vegetables be digested more easily and keep your stomach calm. Chilli is also a great way to boost your metabolism first thing in the morning. This smoothie packs a big punch with super-spice and 'superfood' kale!

Method

Blend all the ingredients (you might want to add ice) together until smooth. Drink immediately.

Serves 2

Ingredients

a small handful of kale leaves (baby kale is good), very finely chopped
2 celery stalks, roughly chopped
1 tsp finely chopped fresh ginger
1 eating apple, cored and chopped
2 carrots, peeled and chopped
½ tsp ground turmeric
½ tsp chilli (red pepper) flakes (optional)
250ml/9fl oz/generous 1 cup water

Super-Boosted Turmeric and Black Pepper Smoothie

394 KCAL

I can't say this enough times – have turmeric every day. A super-spice with so many health benefits, and now research is showing that it could potentially help against dementia. It is good to eat turmeric cooked in food but it may not be fully effective. The advice is to eat turmeric with black pepper, which allows it to be absorbed well by the body. Here is a breakfast smoothie recipe to start your day well.

Method

In a bowl, mix the coconut oil and turmeric together to make a paste. Add it to the other ingredients and blend until smooth. Drink immediately.

Tip

Interchange the vegetables as you like, keeping one 'sweet' vegetable to make it taste good. Add ginger to super-super boost this smoothie!

Serves 2

Ingredients

1 tbsp coconut oil
1 tsp ground turmeric
2 carrots, peeled and chopped
1 avocado, peeled and stoned
75g/2½oz/½cup blueberries
a handful of kale, chopped
200ml/7fl oz/scant 1 cup coconut milk or almond milk
½ tsp freshly ground black pepper

Watermelon, Cinnamon and Cottage Cheese Bowl

Serves 2

Ingredients

10 mint leaves, 6 torn and
   4 reserved to garnish
1 tsp grated fresh ginger
½ tbsp ground cinnamon
600g/1lb 5oz watermelon
   (about ¼ watermelon),
   peeled, deseeded and
   cut into bite-sized pieces
6 tbsp natural cottage cheese
2 tbsp pumpkin seeds, to garnish

This breakfast will challenge your taste buds and make them sing. The freshness of the watermelon and mint combined with the creaminess of the cottage cheese works really well. Ginger adds an edge to the sweetness of the watermelon and will help you start the day with a calm digestion. The cinnamon will keep your glucose levels stable.

Method

In a bowl, combine the mint, ginger and cinnamon. Add the watermelon and mix to combine. Carefully fold in the cottage cheese then leave for a few minutes for all the ingredients to infuse together.

Garnish with the remaining mint leaves and pumpkin seeds.

Tip

As alternatives to watermelon and to 'superfood' your breakfast, use fresh berries like strawberries, raspberries and blueberries. Sprinkle on a little freshly ground black pepper at the end to add an extra zing.

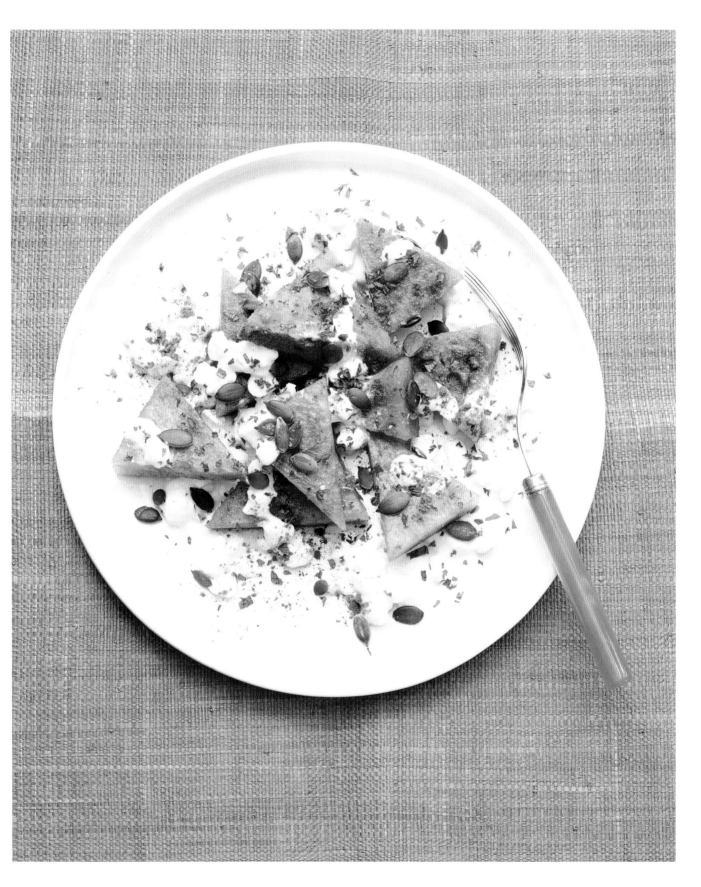

139 KCAL

Middle Eastern Spinach and Egg Stack

Serves 2

Ingredients

½ tsp olive oil for cooking and
   ¼ tsp for greasing the ramekins
100g/3½oz fresh spinach leaves
¼ tsp ground cinnamon
¼ tsp ground coriander
salt and freshly ground
   black pepper
a pinch of chilli (red pepper) flakes
   (optional)
2 tomatoes, sliced into rounds
2 organic eggs
a sprinkling of fresh coriander
   (cilantro) or za'atar, to garnish
   (optional)

A lovely filling but low-fat start to the day, the spinach and tomato are combined with cinnamon and coriander to give a distinctive Middle Eastern flavour. The cinnamon boosts your metabolism and helps keep blood sugar levels stable. The more stable your blood sugar, the less likely you are to overproduce insulin, develop insulin resistance and lay down tummy fat. Coriander seeds are high in vitamin C, great for the digestion and ease any bloating, so will keep you feeling light and healthy all day.

Method

Preheat the oven to 220°C/425°F/Gas mark 7.

Heat the olive oil in a small frying pan. When the oil is hot, add the spinach leaves. When wilted, mix in the cinnamon, coriander, then season well with salt and pepper (add chilli flakes now, if using) and mix together.

Lightly grease 2 ramekins with a little olive oil and place a slice of tomato in each dish. Divide the spinach into 4 equal amounts and spoon a portion into each dish on top of the tomato and press down. Place a second slice of tomato on top of the spinach and top with the rest of the spinach in each ramekin. Crack an egg into each ramekin and place in the hot oven. Cook for 6–8 minutes until the white is set but the yolk is slightly runny.

Gently ease out of the ramekins to serve. Eat with the remaining tomatoes sliced and sprinkled with fresh coriander or za'atar and freshly ground pepper.

Tip

- Increase the health benefits by adding some chilli flakes. Chilli is high in vitamins A and C and is also considered a booster for the metabolism.
- Za'atar is an aromatic mix of herbs and sesame seeds – add this to the cooked egg to bring extra elegance to the dish.

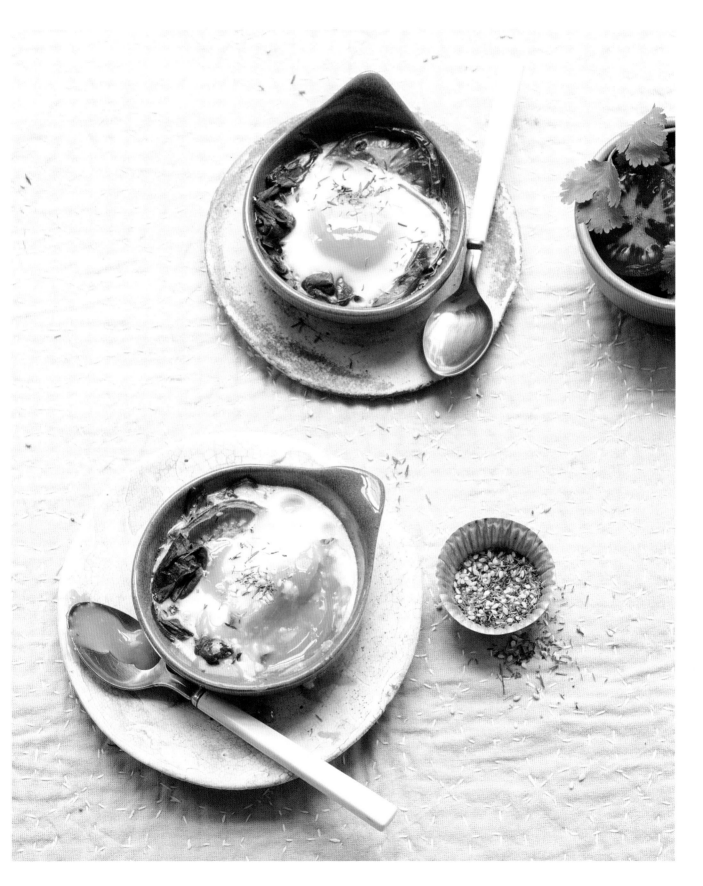

Labneh, Sumac and Fig Breakfast

Serves 2

Ingredients

100g/3½oz/¾ cup mixed berries, blueberries, raspberries, strawberries (slice strawberries, if using)
2 ripe figs, thinly sliced
4 tbsp pomegranate seeds
1 tsp ground sumac
120g/4½oz/½ cup labneh or zero-fat Greek yogurt
½ tbsp runny honey
4–6 walnuts, crushed
8–10 fresh mint leaves, chopped
1 tsp seeds of your choice

We all know that we should eat a balanced breakfast as it stabilises your digestion and will stop you from reaching for those sugary snacks by 11 a.m.! It's important to wake up feeling like you want to eat. This only happens when you get into the habit of eating – so your body will get used to expecting food early in the day. The next step is to prepare breakfasts that you can look forward to and this is one of those. It is colourful, satisfying and a happy, healthy wake-up call, all in one dish! Sumac spice adds a zing and the mint is refreshing and calming. Try using labneh – a yogurt that has been strained to remove all the whey, so the thick, creamy (but low in fat) solids remain. It is eaten in the Middle East for breakfast and in dips, and I like its tangy, rich taste. Add any fruit you like and any seeds – chia seeds, flaxseeds and sunflower seeds all add a higher nutritional value.

Method

Place the fruit in a bowl, sprinkle over the sumac and mint leaves and mix together. Leave to infuse for a few minutes.

In another bowl, mix the labneh with the honey, then top the fruit with the labneh and sprinkle over the crushed nuts and the seeds.

Tips

- Use any seasonal berries you like.
- If you can't find labneh, use Greek yogurt instead.
- To crush the walnuts, place in a tea towel and gently bash with a rolling pin.

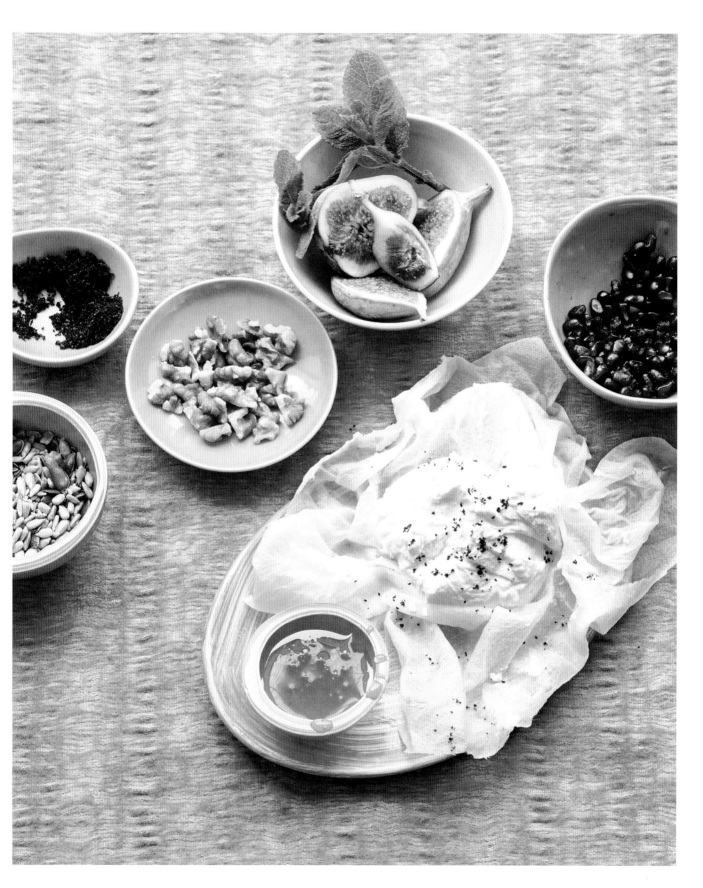

Spicy Veggie Kedgeree

Kedgeree was a dish concocted during the Indian Colonial period – a mixture of rice, fish and eggs – eaten around breakfast time. My version is a spicy and delicious vegetarian lunch or brunch for all the family to share. It uses bulgur wheat instead of rice (bulgur wheat is high in fibre and protein and low in fat, so will keep you full). The spices will energise you throughout the day and the eggs will give you the necessary protein for the start of the day. Using your South Indian Spice Rub, this kedgeree will only take minutes to make and will give you plenty of health benefits from the turmeric (an immune-booster), and cinnamon bark, cloves, dried red chillies, coriander seeds, fenugreek seeds, black cardamom pod, which are all roasted and ground together to help improve health and digestion. I have added cardamom, which has a lovely aroma and soothes the digestion.

Serves 2

Ingredients

2 large free-range eggs
100g/3½oz/½ cup bulgur wheat
 a pinch of chilli (red pepper) flakes
1 tbsp rapeseed (canola) or groundnut (peanut) oil
4 large spring onions (scallions), stems and bulbs, roughly chopped
½ tsp mustard seeds
2 green cardamom pods, bashed lightly to release the flavour
½ tsp South Indian mix (see p.18)
salt
5–6 broccoli florets
30g/1½oz/¼ cup frozen peas
60g/2¼oz fresh baby spinach leaves
a small handful of fresh coriander (cilantro)
a squeeze of fresh lime (optional)

Method

Boil the eggs in a pan for 5–7 minutes until they are hard boiled, then quickly run them under cold water to stop them cooking any further. Set aside.

Cook the bulgur wheat according to the packet instructions but use either vegetable or chicken stock instead of water and add the chilli flakes to the stock. Keep warm.

Heat the oil in a large wok over a high heat. When the oil is very hot, add the white parts of the spring onions, mustard seeds and cardamom pods and as soon as the seeds begin to sizzle, mix in the spice rub and salt and cook for 1 minute.

Add the broccoli florets and the peas and cook until soft (keep the broccoli *al dente*). Wilt in the spinach leaves.

Lightly fork the bulgur wheat so it isn't clumped together, then gently mix into the onion and spice mix. Quarter the eggs and add to the bulgur wheat together with the green parts of the spring onions and coriander leaves. Squeeze over the lime juice (if using) and serve.

Tip

This will work for four people just by doubling the ingredients. I like to eat this with fresh sliced tomatoes and a green salad.

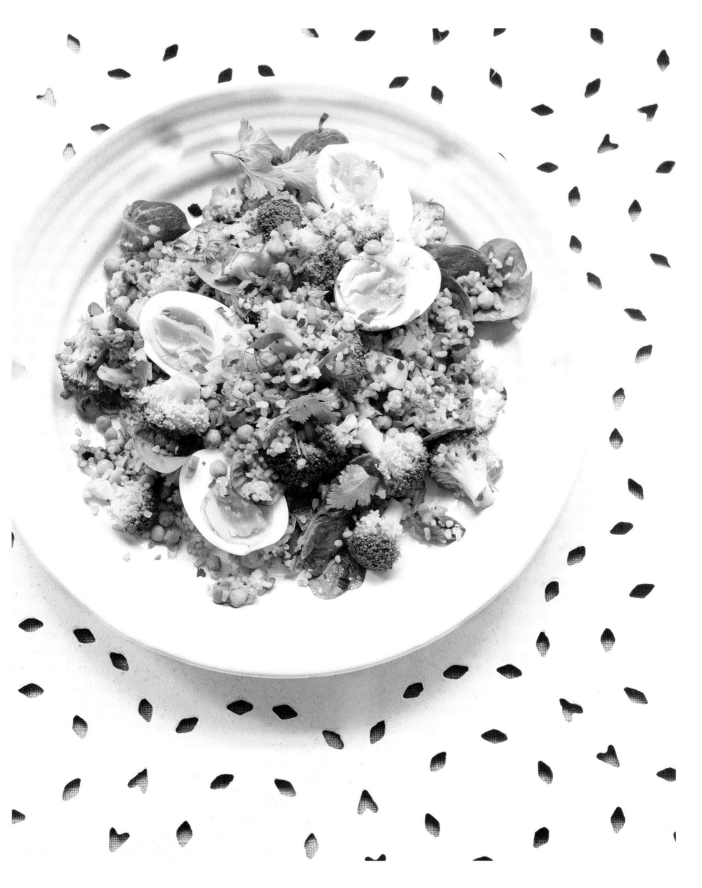

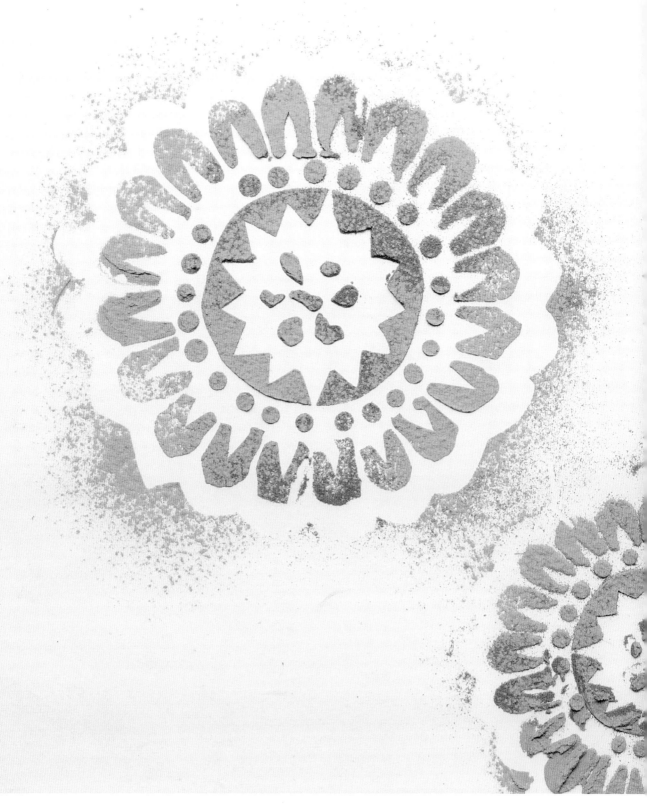

Simple Spicetastic Lunches

What we want to eat for lunch can depend on our mood, how hungry we are and how busy we are. You might want something to fill you up for a long day, something you can make and eat quickly when you are on the go or just a quick snack.

This chapter offers something for every lunch mood: lightly spiced crunchy fresh salads, combining everything from winter fruits and goat's cheese to beetroot and Puy lentils; warming moreish soups from Morocco, India and Thailand; tempting and satisfying quick snacks from tacos to potato cakes to tabbouleh; and more substantial lunches to share with friends such as Chilli Tofu Kebabs with Beetroot and Onion Slaw (p.45), Szechuan Flash-Fried Beef and Citrus Courgettini (p.72) and Energising Japanese Chicken with Edamame Beans and Glass Noodles (p.48).

These lunches will nourish you with vitamins and minerals from the spices and keep you energised for the afternoon ahead.

341 KCAL

Caramelised Pumpkin, Goat's Cheese and Winter Fruit Salad

Serves 2

Ingredients

2 tbsp olive oil
2 tsp cumin seeds
150g/5¼oz pumpkin (cut weight), peeled and cut into 1cm/½in slices or 2.5cm/1in cubes
1 small red onion, peeled and cut into small wedges
½ tbsp ground sumac
salt and freshly ground pepper

For the dressing

juice of ½ large orange (freshly squeezed)
1 tsp Dijon mustard
1 tbsp olive oil
¼ tsp chilli (red pepper) flakes
a pinch of salt, or to taste

For the salad

50g/1¾oz baby spinach
½ a small bag (50g/1¾oz) watercress leaves
2 satsumas, peeled and broken into segments
30g/1oz pomegranate seeds
75g/2¾oz/⅓ cup soft goat's cheese

It's difficult to bring yourself to eat a salad during the winter months, but if you treat your winter vegetables with a dash of spice, you will look forward to eating them. Roast pumpkin with cumin and sumac to give it a caramelised sweet and citrusy taste. Cumin has been attributed special powers as at one time it was thought of as being lucky and helping romance to flourish – a cupid spice! It certainly is a good source of iron and soothes the digestive system.

This is a colourful, versatile and highly nutritious salad with watercress and spinach (full of iron), goat's cheese (protein), pomegranate seeds and satsumas (rich in vitamin C).

Method

Heat 2 tablespoons olive oil in a frying pan over a medium heat. When the oil is hot, add 1 teaspoon cumin seeds and as soon as the seeds start to sizzle add the pumpkin and cook over a gentle heat for 5–7 minutes. Add the onion wedges, season with salt and pepper, then stir in the sumac, turning the vegetables well until they are coated. Gently fry for another 5–6 minutes until the pumpkin and onion are soft and caramelised.

Combine all the ingredients for the dressing and whisk well. Set aside.

Warm a pan over a low heat then add the remaining 1 teaspoon cumin seeds and dry-fry for 3–4 minutes. Take off the heat and grind in a pestle and mortar. Set aside.

Scatter the spinach, watercress leaves, satsuma segments and pomegranate seeds on a plate and place the pumpkin on top. Crumble over the goat's cheese then drizzle over the dressing. Sprinkle the roasted cumin over the top and serve.

Tips

- Use clementines, tangerines or even apples if you prefer instead of satsumas.
- Substitute butternut squash, raw beetroot or sweet potato for the pumpkin if you feel like a change.

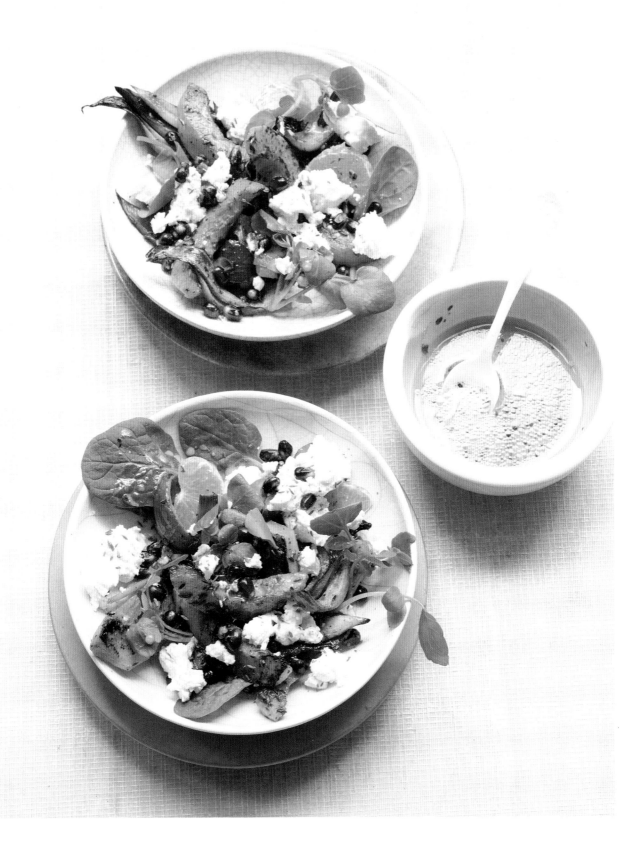

Cumin-Infused Candy Beetroot and Puy Lentil Salad

Serves 2

Ingredients

125g/4½oz/½ cup Puy lentils
1.5 litres/2½ pints/6⅓ cups
    hot water
½ tsp salt
¼ tsp chilli (red pepper) flakes
1 tbsp olive oil
½ tsp cumin seeds
½ small red onion, peeled and
    finely diced
1 garlic clove, peeled and crushed
10 cherry tomatoes, cut in half
¼ tsp salt
freshly ground black pepper
¼ tsp amchoor powder
    or 1 tbsp fresh lemon juice
2 tbsp plain yogurt
¼ small cucumber, finely diced
½ tsp ground cumin
a large handful of rocket (arugula)
2 small candy beetroots or
    2 cooked beetroots (without
    vinegar), sliced into thin rounds
    or thin strips

A salad to feast your eyes and your taste buds – beautiful crispy, sweet rounds of candy beetroot, and soft spiced Puy lentils all topped with an aromatic roasted cumin creamy topping. Nutritious protein-filled lentils, balanced with potassium, magnesium and iron-rich beetroot combined with digestion-calming cumin, this is a perfect energising dish. I have also included a spice called amchoor, which is dried mango powder and has a tart taste, but if you can't find this, then add a tablespoon of lemon juice.

Method

Put the Puy lentils into a medium pan and pour in the hot water. Bring to the boil and add ¼ teaspoon salt and the chilli flakes. Reduce the heat to a simmer and cook for about 15–20 minutes until the lentils are cooked (not too soft and they should retain their shape).

Meanwhile, heat the olive oil in a frying pan over a medium heat. When the oil is hot, add the cumin seeds and cook for 1–2 minutes. Add the onion and garlic, and gently sauté until soft. Add the tomatoes and cook for 2 minutes, then season with salt and pepper.

When the lentils are ready, drain and combine them with the onions and tomatoes and mix thoroughly. (If the lentils are not ready, take the tomato mixture off the heat.) Check the seasoning and stir in the amchoor powder or 1 tablespoon lemon juice. Set aside until the lentils are cool.

Gently whisk the yogurt in a bowl then mix in the cucumber and ground cumin.

Arrange the rocket leaves on a plate and pour over the lentils. Lay the beetroot slices over the top and drizzle over the yogurt mixture. Enjoy!

Tip

This lentil mixture is a good base for lots of salads and will keep for 3–4 days in a refrigerator, so you can make this the day before if wished. Do make a bit extra to add to another salad later in the week. Just double the quantities for four people.

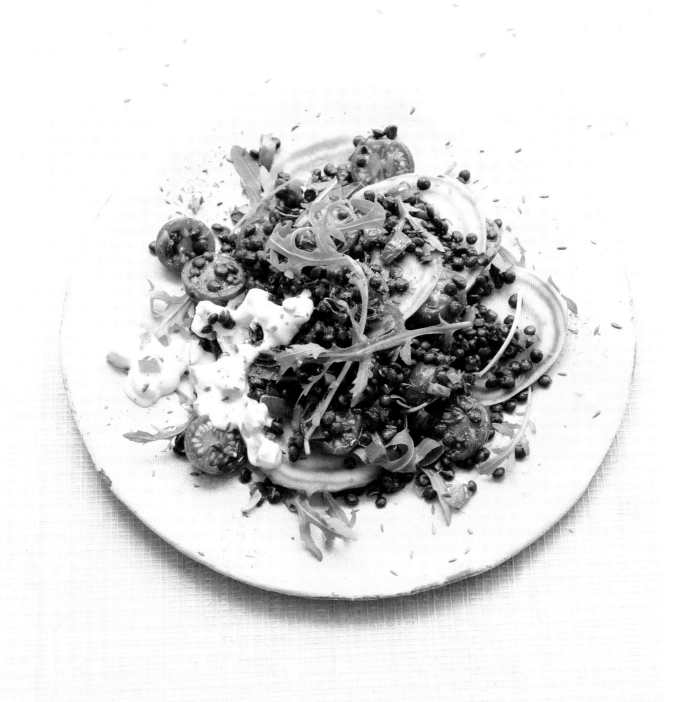

236 KCAL

Vietnamese Chicken and White Cabbage Salad

Serves 2

Ingredients

2 small skinless, boneless chicken breasts
½ tsp olive oil
¼ tsp salt
¼ tsp ground white pepper
¼ white cabbage, very thinly sliced
1 large carrot, peeled and julienned
½ white onion, peeled and very thinly sliced
a small handful of fresh mint leaves
a small handful of fresh coriander (cilantro) leaves
1 tbsp fresh basil leaves (Thai basil leaves, if available, would be perfect)
2 tbsp chopped dry-roasted peanuts

For the salad dressing

1 garlic clove, peeled and finely chopped
½ red chilli, finely chopped
1 tbsp fish sauce
2 tbsp lime juice
1 tsp Shaoxing rice wine

Don't let the name of this salad put you off – it may sound like a boring salad but this is another one of the fantastic salads I discovered in Vietnam and couldn't wait to try out when I returned home. Each mouthful tastes healthy and juicy and simple. Fresh ingredients are brought to life with a sweet and hot dressing. Chilli will get your metabolism moving after lunch and is packed with vitamins and minerals, while garlic will help with blood circulation. This is an altogether healthy, nutritious and low-fat lunch!

Method

Preheat the grill to medium.

Drizzle the chicken breasts with the olive oil and season with the salt and white pepper, then grill for 8–10 minutes on each side (depending on thickness) until cooked through. Cut the chicken into thin slices and set aside.

In a large bowl, combine the cabbage, carrots, onions and herbs. In another bowl, mix together all the ingredients for the dressing, then pour the dressing onto the vegetables and toss well. Place the sliced chicken on top and garnish with the roasted peanuts.

Tips

- Slice the vegetables as thinly as possible (almost julienne).
- For a vegetarian option, use portobello mushrooms or silken tofu instead of chicken.

Chilli Tofu Kebabs with Beetroot and Onion Slaw

264 KCAL

Firm tofu is packed with nutrients but I find that it needs a bit of help with flavour. However, it does soak up flavours well, so if you add some spices, you will not only gain goodness from in the tofu, but also from the spices! I use my Tandoori Spice Rub for this recipe as it adds the benefits of iron-rich cumin, anti-inflammatory properties from the turmeric and a metabolism kick from the chilli.

Method

If using wooden skewers, then presoak 4 wooden skewers in a bowl of water before using to prevent them burning under the grill.

To make the beetroot slaw, mix the lemon and honey together and season with the salt and pepper. Put the beetroot, onion, apple and carrot in a bowl and stir in the lemon and honey mixture. Sprinkle over the ground cumin.

Preheat the grill to medium.

In a bowl, combine the yogurt with ½ tablespoon Tandoori Spice Rub, lemon juice and ½ tablespoon of olive oil. Add salt to taste then gently add the tofu pieces and stir until the tofu is coated with the yogurt mixture.

Put the courgette and the pepper pieces in another bowl and season with the rest of the spice rub and salt and pepper. Pour the remaining olive oil on the vegetables and mix thoroughly.

Shake the yogurt mixture off the tofu. Thread the tofu and vegetables alternatively onto the skewers and grill for about 8–10 minutes until cooked. Keep basting the tofu with the remaining yogurt mixture and turn the skewers halfway through cooking.

Tips

• This is a light vegetarian dish but it would work well with chicken breast pieces or fish.
• Make the beetroot slaw first so that the flavours can meld together.

Serves 2

Ingredients

For the tofu kebabs

2 tbsp plain yogurt
1 tbsp Tandoori Spice Rub (see p.18)
1 tsp lemon juice
1 tbsp olive oil
¼ tsp salt
freshly ground black pepper
150g/5¼oz firm tofu, cut into cubes
1 large courgette (zucchini), sliced into thick rounds
1 red (bell) pepper, deseeded and cut into cubes
a small handful of fresh coriander (cilantro)

For the beetroot and onion slaw

2 tbsp lemon juice
a drizzle of honey
a pinch of salt and pepper
1 medium beetroot, grated or thinly sliced
½ red onion, peeled and very thinly sliced
1 apple, cored and grated
1 carrot, peeled and grated or finely sliced
¾ tsp ground cumin

Fresh Herb Maroque Tabbouleh with Minted Halloumi

Serves 2

Ingredients

½ red or yellow (bell) pepper,
    deseeded and cut into
    thin strips
1 small (zucchini) courgette,
    cut into very small cubes
60g/2¼oz halloumi, cut into strips
1½ tbsp olive oil
½ tsp dried mint
½ tsp chilli flakes
100g/3½oz/½ cup bulgur wheat
1 tsp Moroccan Spice Rub
    (see p.19)
2 tbsp lemon juice
100g/3½oz cherry or small vine
    tomatoes, roughly chopped
2 spring onions (scallions),
    finely chopped
28g/1oz fresh flat-leaf parsley,
    leaves only, roughly chopped
28g/1oz fresh mint, leaves only,
    roughly chopped
salt

A sprinkle of my Moroccan Spice Rub will bring this salad to life with a delicious sweet spicy taste and the wonderful aroma from the cumin, cinnamon and coriander. The Moroccan Spice Rub includes spices containing vitamins and minerals which aid health and digestion. This tabbouleh salad is packed with fresh herbs and I love adding grilled salty halloumi to add some protein and complement the lightness of the herbs. I have also added pepper and courgette, which are not traditional in tabbouleh, but these add colour to the salad and make it a more filling lunch.

Method

Preheat the grill to medium.

Drizzle the pepper, courgette and halloumi slices with ½ tablespoon olive oil, the dried mint and chilli flakes, and place on a grill tray under the grill. Cook for 4–5 minutes until the pepper is soft and the halloumi is tinged brown.

Cook the bulgur wheat according to the packet instructions. While still warm, mix in the Moroccan Spice Rub, the olive oil and lemon juice, then mix in the pepper and courgette. After 2–3 minutes (as the bulgur wheat cools), add the tomatoes, spring onion, parsley and mint, and mix well. Season with salt. Place the halloumi slices over the top of the salad and serve.

Tips

• This salad will keep in the refrigerator for 2–3 days.
• It also goes well with other cheese such as feta or cottage cheese. Just double the ingredients for four people.

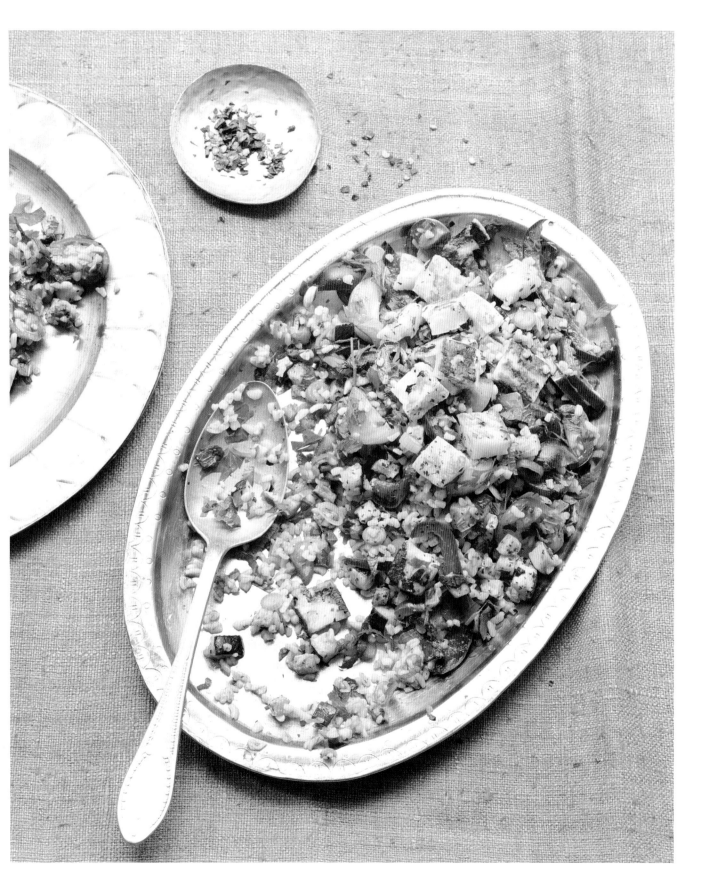

435 KCAL

Energising Japanese Chicken with Edamame Beans and Glass Noodles

Serves 2

Ingredients

1 medium skinless, boneless chicken breast, cut into very thin slices
100g/3½oz glass noodles
1 red (bell) pepper, cored, deseeded and sliced into thin strips
1 carrot, peeled and thinly sliced
6 small radishes, thinly sliced
2 spring onions (scallions), cut into small chunks
100g/3½oz edamame beans
1 tbsp toasted sesame seeds (optional)

For the dressing

1 garlic clove, peeled and finely chopped
1 thumb-sized piece fresh ginger, peeled and finely grated
1 medium red chilli, finely chopped
½ small bunch of fresh coriander (cilantro), save a few leaves to garnish, roughly chopped
2 tbsp soy sauce
1 tbsp orange juice
2 tbsp mirin or rice wine vinegar
2 tsp fish sauce
½ tsp salt
½ tsp sesame oil

This is a light, super-healthy, fresh salad but the addition of the noodles and beans give it texture and make it a filling lunch. You will feel good and satisfied after eating it. Glass noodles are healthier than wheat noodles and are made from green beans, broad beans, and peas, which also makes them gluten-free and a source of iron, calcium, and fibre. They are opaque until soaked in water.

The ginger in this salad will help your digestion, while the garlic cleanses and the chilli adds heat to get your metabolism on the go. I love this salad and could eat it every day!

Method

To make the dressing, put the garlic, ginger, chilli and coriander in a saucepan and pour in the soy sauce, orange juice, mirin, fish sauce, salt and sesame oil. Stir the chicken slices into the dressing and simmer over a gentle heat for 4–5 minutes, or until the chicken is poached and cooked through, taking care not to let it boil. Take off the heat and set aside.

Cook the noodles according to the packet instructions, usually about 15–20 minutes, but they do vary as some only need soaking.

Drain the noodles and tip into a large bowl. Mix through the red pepper, carrot, radishes, spring onions and edamame beans. Pour over the dressing and chicken and mix through. Garnish with coriander leaves and toasted sesame seeds.

Tips

• You can buy toasted sesame seeds, or I toast them in a dry frying pan over a medium heat for 4–5 minutes until lightly brown. Keep moving them so they don't burn.
• For a vegetarian option, use a firm tofu marinated in soy sauce and chilli flakes and add more of the vegetables.

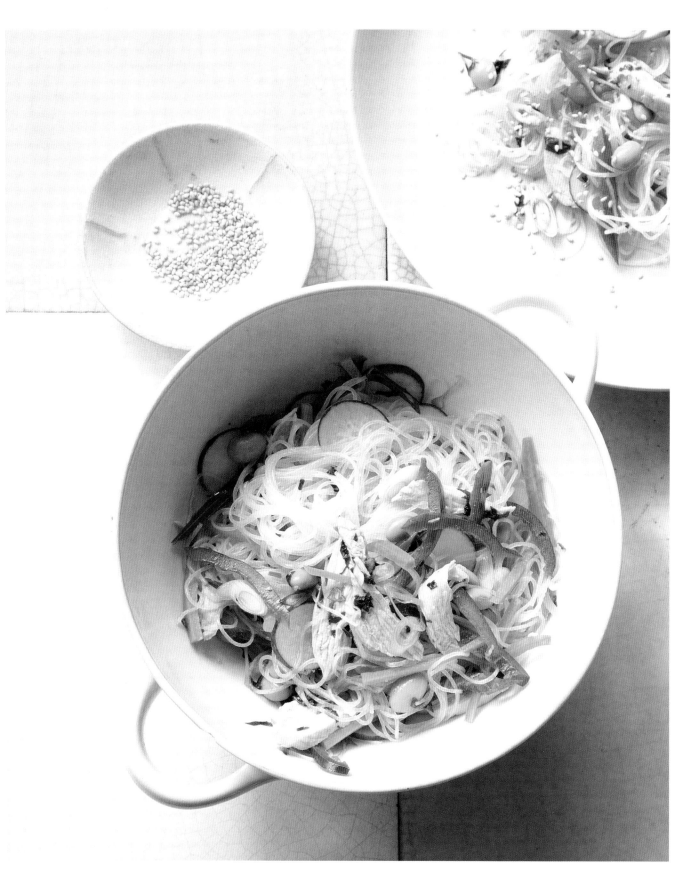

287 KCAL

Fajita-Style Chicken with Papaya and Kiwi Relish

Serves 2

Ingredients

For the chicken

2 skinless, boneless chicken breast
fillets, washed and patted dry
1 heaped tsp Mexican Spice Rub
(see p.18)
juice of ½ lime
¼ tsp salt
1 tbsp olive oil

For the relish

1 large ripe (but not too soft)
papaya, peeled and finely diced
2 kiwi fruits, peeled and
finely chopped
½ red (bell) pepper, finely diced
1 spring onion, finely chopped
¼ small red chilli
8–10 fresh mint leaves,
finely sliced
juice of ½ lime
½ tsp olive oil
2–3 grinds of black pepper
a pinch of salt

Bring a little Mexican flavour into your lunch with this griddled chicken simply marinated in a mixture of the Mexican Spice Rub and lime juice. A low-fat dish, it packs a punch in flavour and in health. Serve the chicken with the beautiful, colourful and sweet-and-spicy Papaya and Kiwi Relish. Papaya has been called the 'fruit of the angels', as it's lush in colour and rich in vitamins A and C. Kiwi fruit has one of the highest contents of vitamin C. *Relish illustrated on p.57.*

Method

Place the chicken breasts between 2 pieces of clingfilm and, using a mallet, pound them until they are a medium thickness all over. Using a sharp knife, score deep lines into the chicken (don't go all the way through the chicken) then cut into 2.5cm/1in strips. Put the chicken in a bowl, rub the Mexican Spice Rub all over the chicken, then pour most of the lime juice over. Cover and set aside while making the relish.

In a bowl, mix together the papaya and kiwi, then gently mix in the red pepper, spring onion, chilli and mint. Pour over the lime juice and olive oil, season with the salt and pepper, and mix again.

Heat a griddle pan and brush with the olive oil. Lay the chicken pieces across the griddle and cook over a medium heat for 4–5 minutes each side, brushing halfway through with any lime juice that's left, until the chicken is cooked. Squeeze a little more lime juice over the chicken when serving.

Tip

This recipe can be up-scaled to a lovely dinner by doubling all the ingredients.

Immunising Tasty Turmeric Soup

267
KCAL

For as long as I can remember, my family has used turmeric both as a spice in food and for medicinal purposes. In India it has been used for centuries as a medicinal herb and now in the West, studies are showing the health benefits of turmeric. Turmeric contains a compound called curcumin, which has been shown to calm pain and inflammation. It is also anti-fungal, antibacterial, antiviral and a powerful antioxidant, so, altogether, it's a great way of keeping your body immunised against illness. Feel the goodness flowing into your body as you eat this soup – turmeric combines with hearty pearl barley, and earthy vegetables – leeks, carrots and mushrooms – and the other super-spices ginger and garlic.

Method

Preheat the oven to 180°C/350°F/Gas mark 4.

Heat the olive oil in an ovenproof saucepan or heavy-based casserole over a medium heat. Add the leeks, ginger and garlic, and sauté for 3–4 minutes, or until soft. Add the turmeric, paprika and bay leaf, mix and add the barley and vegetables. Turn in the spices then pour in the stock and bring to the boil.

Place the saucepan in the hot oven and cook for 30 minutes. Check there is enough liquid (if not, add a small cup of hot water or stock and return to the oven).

After 30 minutes, sprinkle in the coriander and parsley. Check the seasoning and add salt and pepper if needed.

Tips
- To make this a dinner soup, just double the quantities.
- For an even healthier option, add some chopped kale at the end.

Serves 2

Ingredients

2 tbsp olive oil
1 medium leek, finely chopped
1cm/½in piece fresh ginger, peeled and finely chopped
1 large garlic clove, peeled and finely chopped
1 tsp ground turmeric
½ tsp paprika
1 dried bay leaf
30g/1oz/scant ¼ cup pearl barley, rinsed
1 carrot, diced
2 celery stalks, diced
3–4 chestnut (cremini) mushrooms, cut in half then thinly sliced
600ml/1 pint/2½ cups hot low-salt chicken or vegetable stock (broth)
a small handful of fresh coriander (cilantro), roughly chopped
a small handful of chopped fresh parsley
salt and freshly ground black pepper

Hot and Fragrant Tom Yam Soup

Serves 4

Ingredients

10–12 large raw prawns (shrimp),
    head and shells left on
1 tbsp olive oil
3 shallots, peeled and finely diced
5cm/2in piece galangal or fresh
    ginger, peeled and thinly sliced
a large handful of fresh coriander
    (cilantro), stems and leaves
    separated and stems
    roughly chopped
2 lemongrass stalks, pounded
    gently, peeled outer skin off,
    broken in the middle and then
    in half
1.2 litres/2 pints/5 cups hot
    low-salt chicken stock (broth)
3 kaffir lime leaves, scrunched up
    in your hand (this will release
    the flavour)
2–3 bird's eye chillies, or
    according to taste, sliced down
    the middle but keep whole
½ tsp palm sugar
1 tbsp light soy sauce
2 tsp nam pla or fish sauce
juice of 1 lime
100g/3½oz pak choi,
    roughly sliced

Sweet, sour, hot and very low in fat – both a fantastically tasty and virtuous soup. The chillies will give a big jolt to your metabolism and to your taste buds! The galangal will soothe your digestive system and get your blood circulating well. I remember the first time I tasted Thai food – delicate aromas, keen flavours and a lavishness of freshness. My Tom Yam soup is a fragrant broth that my lovely son Ben and I cook when we want something warm and spicy to fuel us, keep us healthy and make a few sweat beads appear on our foreheads!

Method

Peel the prawns, reserving the shells, and crush the prawn heads. Set the prawns aside.

Heat the oil in a saucepan over a medium-high heat. Add the prawn heads, shells, shallot, ginger or galangal, coriander stems and lemongrass stalks and fry for 2–3 minutes. Pour in the chicken stock then add the kaffir lime leaves, chillies and palm sugar. Bring to the boil, then reduce the heat and simmer gently for 8–10 minutes.

Strain the soup to remove the prawn shells, prawn heads and the lemongrass (and the chillies if you want), then pour the soup back into the pan. Mix in the soy sauce, nam pla (fish sauce) and lime juice, then add the prawns and pak choi and cook for 2–3 minutes, or until the prawns are cooked. Sprinkle over the coriander leaves, then taste and add a little more soy sauce if required. Serve.

Tips

This recipe uses prawns but you can make a vegetarian version with mushrooms, water chestnuts, pak choi or choi sam, adding tofu for protein. Bird's eye chillies are very hot so adjust the amount to your taste.

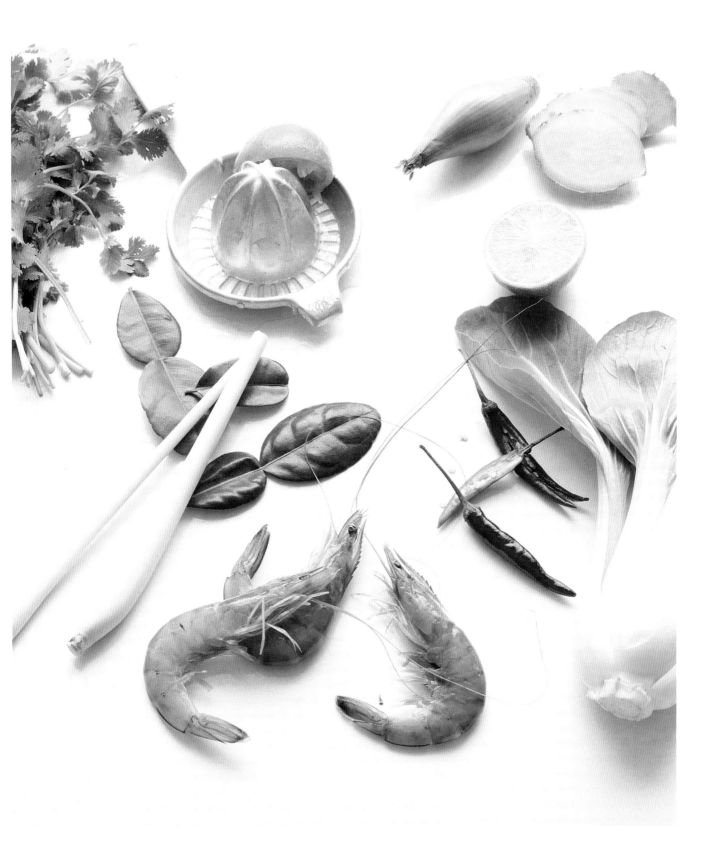

Indian Reviving Tomato Shorba

Serves 2

Ingredients

2 tbsp olive oil
1 tsp finely chopped fresh ginger
1 garlic clove, peeled and finely chopped
½ small green chilli, finely chopped
1 dried or fresh bay leaf
¼ tsp salt
8 large vine red fresh tomatoes, roughly chopped
140ml/5fl oz/scant ⅔ cup hot water

For the tempering

½ tsp cumin seeds
¼ tsp black mustard seeds
5–6 fresh curry leaves
½ tsp ground turmeric
½ tsp ground coriander
¼ tsp chilli powder
a small handful of fresh coriander (cilantro) leaves, roughly chopped

This is the vegetarian Indian equivalent of Jewish chicken soup, or Jewish penicillin as it's commonly called as it is given at any sign of a cold or any illness! In this version, there is no chicken but it is the spices that will keep you warm in the winter and keep colds at bay. Tempering the spices (cumin, turmeric, ground coriander and mustard seeds) at the end lift this soup's taste and health properties. A light, easy, very low-fat rejuvenating soup, cook this slowly, make double and store in the refrigerator for a few days, then feel it reviving you as you eat it. If you are making double, temper the spices when you serve the soup.

Method

Heat the oil in a saucepan over a medium heat. When the oil is hot, add the ginger and garlic and cook for 1 minute. Add the chilli, bay leaf, salt and fresh tomatoes, mix and cook for a further 2–3 minutes. Pour in the hot water. Bring to the boil, then reduce the heat and simmer for 15–20 minutes. The tomatoes should be completely mashed up but there should still be some liquid in the pan.

Either strain the tomatoes through a sieve until you are left with just the liquid and pour into a saucepan. Or blend with a hand-held blender until smooth. If the soup is too thick, add a little more hot water.

To temper the spices, heat the oil in a small pan over a medium heat. When the oil is hot, add the cumin seeds, mustard seeds and the curry leaves (if using). When these all start to crackle, quickly add the turmeric, ground coriander and salt to taste. As everything sizzles, pour over the tomato soup and mix in lightly. Mix in the chopped coriander and serve immediately.

Tips

• Add precooked chicken pieces at the end if you want to add some protein to this soup. The curry leaves add a distinctive flavour but if you can't get them, just leave them out.
• This recipe can easily be doubled for four people.

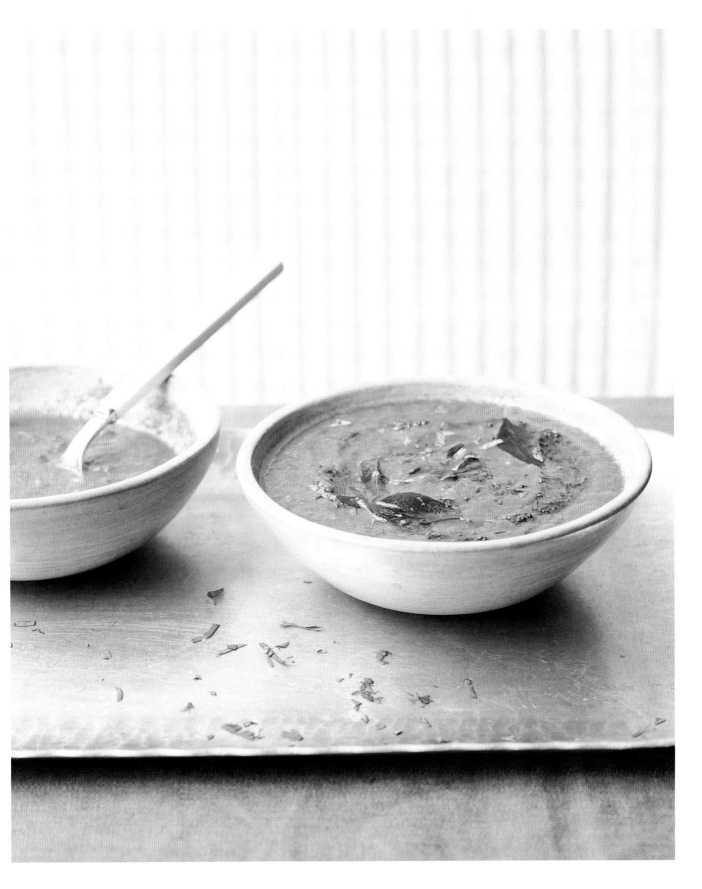

138 KCAL

Hara Bhara Kebabs (Healthy Sweet Potato and Spinach Cakes)

**Serves 4
(makes 8 kebabs)**

Ingredients

1 large sweet potato (about 600 g/1lb 5oz), peeled and cut into small cubes
salt and freshly ground black pepper
75g/2½oz spinach leaves, very finely chopped
45g/1½oz/⅓ cup cooked frozen peas
½ green chilli, finely chopped
½ tsp red chilli powder
1 tsp finely chopped fresh ginger
¼ tsp salt, or to taste
1 tsp ground turmeric
½ tsp ground cumin
a large handful of fresh coriander (cilantro) leaves, roughly chopped
2 tbsp olive oil
1–2 tbsp plain (all-purpose) flour, for dusting

Tips

- These patties will keep for 3–4 days covered in the refrigerator so cook a few extra for another meal.
- For your extra-hungry days, you can eat these stuffed in a wholemeal pitta pocket with the raita drizzled over.

Hara bhara kebabs are a delicious street food in North India – it literally means, kebabs stuffed with green ingredients. These vegetarian patties are normally made from potato, but I have substituted sweet potato as it has a low glycaemic index (GI). This means that it will release energy steadily and will keep you feeling fuller longer. It also adds a nice sweet balance to the spices. I have upscaled the spices to make these extra healthy and tasty. Ginger will keep the digestion working well and adds a quiet 'heat' and turmeric is an extra addition of mine as it's a great antiseptic aid for the body. I like to eat these with a Cucumber and Mint Raita (see p.143) as the yogurt provides valuable protein. *Also shown, Papaya and Kiwi Relish (see p.50).*

Method

Preheat the oven to 200°C/400°F/Gas mark 6.

Place the diced sweet potatoes on a baking tray and season with a few grinds of salt and pepper. Cook in the oven for 10 minutes, or until soft. Take out of the oven and leave to cool. Leave the oven on.

Place the spinach leaves in a saucepan with just the water from washing clinging to the leaves and heat gently until they are cooked. Drain off any excess water.

In a large bowl, place the peas, spinach and sweet potato and mash lightly with a fork. Add the remaining ingredients, except the oil, and mix well until smooth. If the mixture is a bit sticky and wet, add 1 teaspoon plain flour. Dust your hands lightly with flour then divide the mixture into 8 equal portions and flatten into medium-sized cakes. Place the patties on a baking tray. Drizzle the oil over the top and cook in the hot oven for 5–6 minutes on each side until crisp and cooked. Alternatively, grill the patties on a high heat for 3–4 minutes on each side.

Serve with wholemeal pitta pockets stuffed with crisp lettuce and a cool Cucumber and Mint Raita (see p.143).

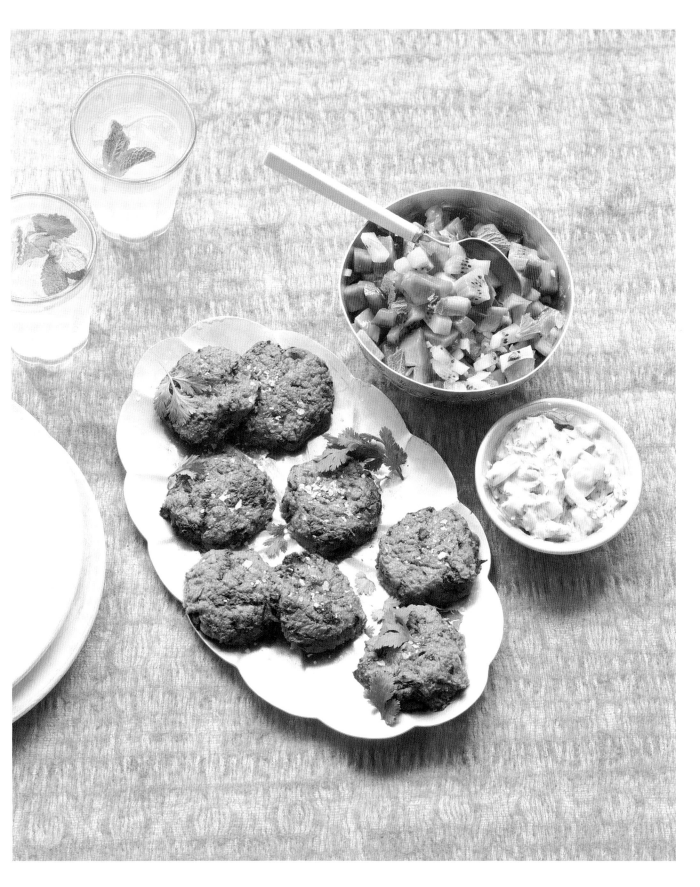

Keralan Masala Fish with Spinach and Pomegranate Raita

Serves 2

Ingredients

For the fish

2 white fish fillets, either tilapia
   or red snapper
½ tbsp South Indian Spice Rub
   (see p.18)
1 tbsp lemon juice
¼ tsp cornflour
salt
2 tsp olive oil

For the raita

1 tsp olive oil
100g/3½oz baby spinach
25g/1oz fresh watercress,
   finely chopped
150g/5¼oz/⅔ cup plain yogurt
a small handful of fresh coriander
   (cilantro), roughly chopped
½ tsp roasted ground cumin
a pinch of freshly ground
   black pepper
25g/1oz pomegranate seeds

South Indians love their fish. They coat it with flavourful spices and either deep-fry or shallow-fry it. In this recipe, it is lightly grilled and is quick and easy to make with my South Indian Spice Rub. My spice rub includes fenugreek and turmeric. Turmeric can offer relief from pain and inflammation and guards against bacterial infections, while fenugreek can lower blood sugar due to its high fibre content. The spinach and pomegranate are packed with protein, calcium from the yogurt, and the spinach and watercress are packed with iron to give you an energy boost. Make the raita thick and it will be filling.

Method

Score the fish lightly on both sides.

Mix the spice rub, lemon juice, cornflour and salt to taste together in a large bowl. Add the fish and turn the fish until it is coated well in the spices. Cover and set aside for 10–15 minutes while making the raita.

In a non-stick frying pan, heat the olive oil over a medium heat. Add the spinach and the watercress and cook for 2–3 minutes until wilted. Take off the heat and leave to cool, then discard any excess water.

Put the yogurt in a large bowl and whisk gently until smooth. Mix in the spinach, watercress and coriander. Sprinkle with a few grinds of black pepper and the ground cumin and drop in the pomegranate seeds.

When the raita is ready, heat the grill to medium. Drizzle the fish with the olive oil and grill the fish until cooked, about 3–4 minutes on each side.

Serve the raita with the fish.

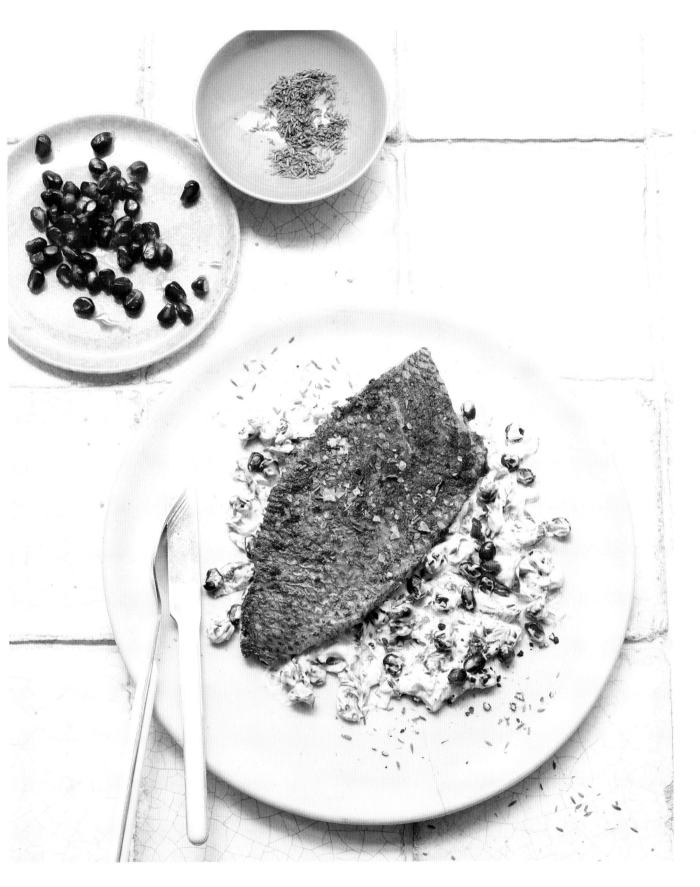

328 KCAL

Mexicana Bean Tacos

Serves 2

Ingredients

2 tbsp olive oil

½ small red onion, peeled and finely chopped

1 garlic clove, peeled and finely minced

¾ tbsp Mexican Spice Rub (see p.18)

¼ tsp salt

½ can (200g/7oz) kidney beans, drained and rinsed

¼ red or green (bell) pepper, deseeded and cut into very small cubes

70g/2½oz/scant ⅔ cup canned sweetcorn, drained and rinsed

1 spring onion (scallion), roughly chopped

4–6 cherry tomatoes, cut into quarters

3 tbsp lime juice and a squeeze for the garnish

½ avocado, peeled and cut into small chunks

a small handful of fresh coriander (cilantro) leaves

6–8 lettuce leaves (iceberg lettuce is good)

1 carrot, peeled and finely grated

Use your Mexican Spice Rub to create a quick and nutritious light, tasty lunch. All the flavours of Mexico – beans, avocados, chipotle chillies and sweetcorn (corn is king in so many parts of Mexico) are combined in this dish. Lettuce is used here as a 'wrap' or 'spoon' as it provides a low-fat and fresh alternative to wheat wraps and it's also gluten free. This unassuming dish is low-carb and includes protein and a spice mix that provides plenty of health benefits – cumin and coriander are high in iron, while manganese, magnesium and coriander are especially good for the digestion. So, after eating this light lunch, you should feel good all day.

Method

Heat the olive oil in a pan over a medium heat. Add the onion and garlic, season with the Mexican Spice Rub and salt, and cook for 1–2 minutes. Add the beans, red or green pepper and sweetcorn, and turn in the mixture for 2–3 minutes. Take the pan off the heat.

In a bowl, mix together the spring onion, tomatoes and lime juice, then gently fold in the avocado. Add this mixture to the beans and corn and sprinkle with the coriander. Divide the mixture between the wraps and top with a few sticks of grated carrot on each. Squeeze over some lime juice to serve.

Tips

- Use other combinations of beans if you prefer, such as black beans or pinto beans. Black olives are good too, as are a few slices of jalapeño chillies for a change.
- This makes four lettuce tacos per person, but you can double the ingredients for four people.

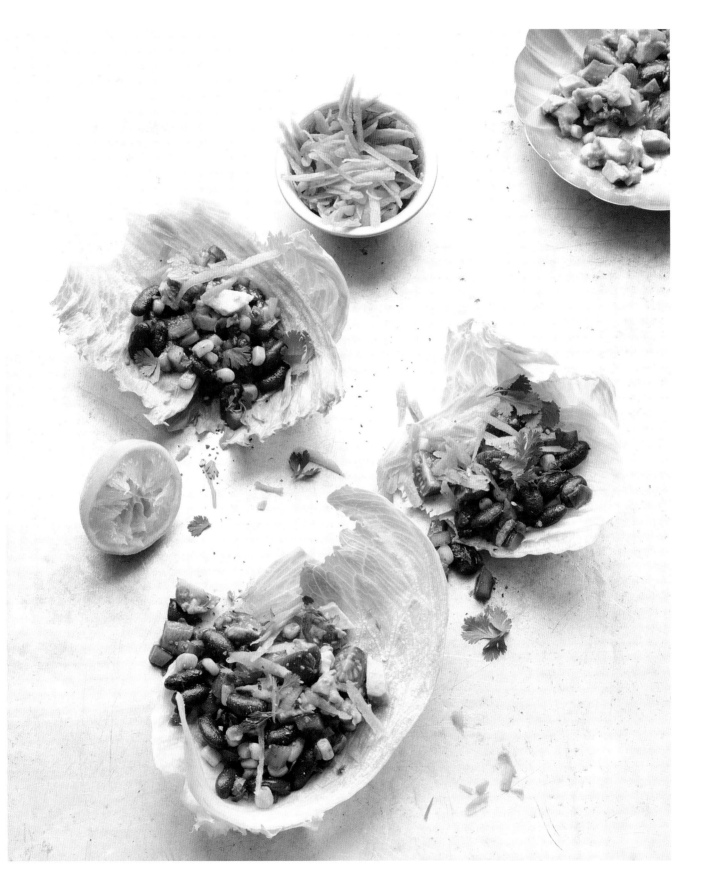

150 KCAL

My Super-Herby Feel-Good Frittata

Serves 4

Ingredients

2 tbsp olive oil

2 garlic cloves, peeled and finely chopped

4 spring onions (scallions), roughly chopped

1 tbsp Mediterranean Spice Rub (see p.19)

100g/3½oz baby spinach leaves, roughly chopped

50g/1¾oz watercress, roughly chopped

a small handful of fresh thyme leaves

a few fresh mint leaves, finely chopped

5–6 large organic eggs

1 tbsp milk (optional)

salt and freshly ground black pepper

The Mediterranean Spice Rub is so versatile and adds sunny flavours to so many dishes. I love making a frittata that is stuffed full of herbs and green vegetables. The protein from the eggs, the goodness from the spice mix – dried oregano, thyme, chilli and paprika – with the fresh herbs and garlic gives you a balanced, wholly nutritious meal. Thyme contains vitamins and minerals and is rich in antioxidants. The word 'oregano' comes from the Greek words *oros* and *ganos* which means mountain and joy (so a happy herb from the mountains!). Oregano contains minerals and vitamin K, which is essential in keeping our bones strong. Both oregano and thyme contain the essential oil thymol, which is known to have antibacterial and anti-fungal properties, and the spinach and watercress leaves really tip the health scales.

Method

Preheat the oven to 180°C/350°F/Gas mark 4.

In an ovenproof medium non-stick frying pan with high sides, heat 1 tablespoon olive oil over a medium heat. Add the garlic and spring onions and cook gently for 3–4 minutes. Mix in the Mediterranean Spice Rub, then add the spinach and watercress leaves and cook for 2 minutes. Mix in the fresh herbs then take off the heat and cool slightly.

Break the eggs into a large bowl and add the milk (if using). Beat the eggs then season well with salt and pepper. Add the herb and vegetable mixture to the eggs and mix lightly.

Heat the frying pan over a medium-low heat and add the remaining olive oil. When the oil is hot, pour in the egg mixture and shake the pan gently so the egg covers the base. Place the frying pan in the oven and cook for 5–8 minutes until the egg is set and cooked through.

Tips

- You can make this for two people and eat it over two days or make it for four as this is a lovely sharing dish.
- Use any green leaves in this recipe – wild rocket and lambs lettuce leaves are good.
- Eat with a fresh green salad or if eating for dinner, with my Shirazi Salad (see p.136).

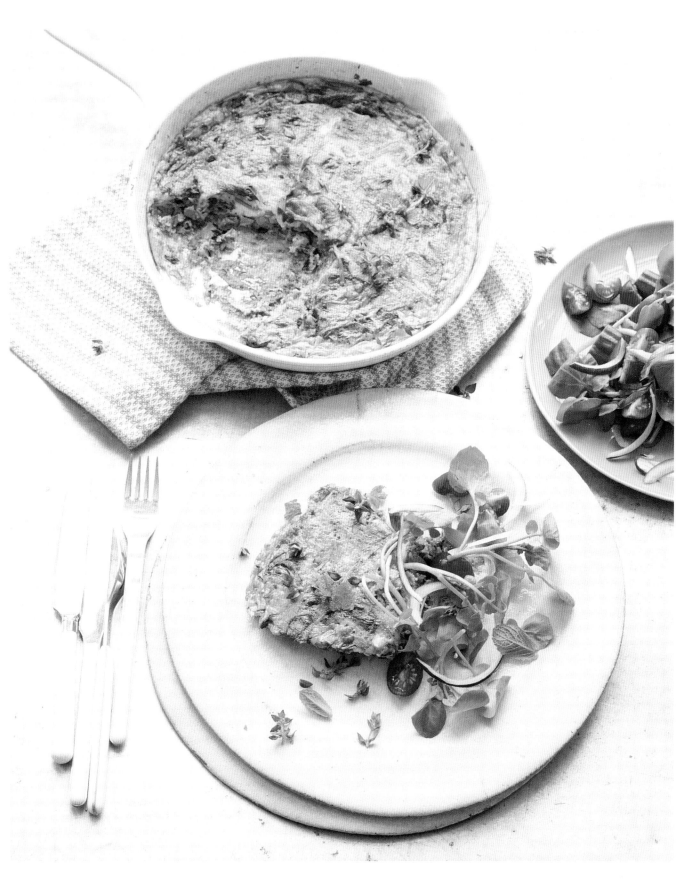

392 KCAL

Revitalising Superfoods Salad with Farro

Serves 2

Ingredients

30g/1oz pearled farro
85g/3oz broccoli florets
1 medium cooked beetroot, chopped into small cubes
½ avocado, peeled and diced
28g/1oz baby kale leaves, roughly chopped
¼ red onion, peeled and finely chopped
a small handful of fresh basil, leaves only, roughly chopped
40g/1½oz/scant ¼ cup soft goat's cheese, crumbled
½ tsp ground cumin
2 tbsp pumpkin seeds (optional)

For the dressing

1 tbsp olive oil
2 tbsp lemon juice (about ½ lemon)
½ tsp Dijon mustard
½ tsp ground sumac
salt and freshly ground black pepper

You will fall in love with this salad and will want to eat it every day, so make up a large amount! It is satisfying, energising and invigorating and will give your digestion a boost to make you feel good all day! Farro is an ancient grain, which is commonly eaten in Italy. It has a lovely nutty taste and has a low glycaemic index (GI). It is high in fibre to stabilise blood sugar levels and will help you feel full for longer. The sumac adds a zing and is high in antioxidants, while the roasted cumin will keep your digestion calm and working smoothly. The soft goat's cheese adds the low-fat protein to this dish. In short, everything in this salad is good for you!

Method

Cook the farro according to the packet instructions. Set aside.

Steam the broccoli until *al dente*, then plunge into cold water to retain its colour. Allow to cool and dry.

Make the dressing by placing all the ingredients in a jar, sealing with a lid and shaking vigorously. Set aside.

Combine the beetroot, broccoli, avocado, kale and onion with the basil leaves in a bowl. Pour over the dressing and mix well.

Fold the farro into the salad, then crumble over the goat's cheese and sprinkle over the ground cumin and pumpkin seeds.

Tips

• You can substitute the goat's cheese for feta cheese, if you prefer.
• Buy pearled or semi-pearled farro as this will cook more quickly than the unprocessed version.
• Double the quantities for 4 people.

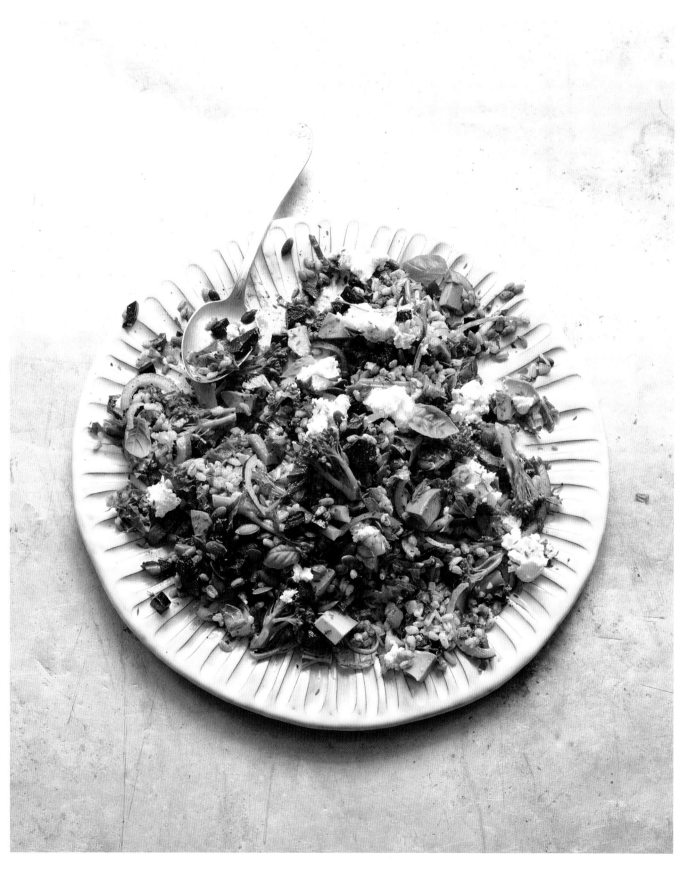

214 KCAL

Serves 2

Ingredients

For the dressing

1 tsp finely diced fresh ginger
¼ tsp salt
a small handful of fresh coriander (cilantro), stems and leaves
3 tbsp lime juice
½ tsp Szechuan-Style Spice Rub (see p.19)
1 tbsp soy sauce
1 tsp runny honey
1 small red chilli, finely chopped

For the salad

3 medium carrots, peeled and grated or shredded
½ red (bell) pepper, thinly sliced
3 celery stalks, finely diced
½ small red onion, peeled and very finely sliced or finely diced
a small bunch of fresh coriander (cilantro) leaves (save the stems for the dressing)
20g/¾oz/scant ¼ cup cashew nuts (not salted or roasted)
1 tbsp toasted sesame seeds

Super-Crunchy Asian Salad

It's official – I just love Thai salads. This salad is so crunchy, crisp and each mouthful feels like it is revitalising you and setting you up for the afternoon. The textures are great – raw sweet carrots, crispy celery, gentle-biting red onions, red pepper, clean fresh herbs topped with crunchy cashew nuts, all enveloped in a zingy, aromatic spice dressing. You can eat this on its own as a low-fat lunch or with an oily mackerel fillet or sliced grilled chicken breast. On my indulgent days, I have been known to eat this with a generous dollop of white crabmeat – divine! The Asian dressing of coriander, chilli, soy sauce, ginger and lime juice with a hit of my Szechuan-Style Spice Rub will give the simple salad ingredients a complex taste!

Method

To make the dressing, pound the ginger with the salt and coriander stems in a pestle and mortar (you can also use a food processor) to make a smooth paste. Add the remaining dressing ingredients and mix thoroughly.

In a large bowl, combine all the salad ingredients, except the cashew nuts and sesame seeds. Pour the dressing over the salad and toss together. Check the seasoning, then sprinkle over the cashew nuts and sesame seeds and serve.

Tips

- Substitute edamame beans for the cashew nuts to make this salad even lower in fat but still crunchy.
- Green papaya is also wonderful in this salad if you can find it.
- This dressing will keep for 2–3 days and works with many raw food salads.
- You can buy toasted sesame seeds, or I toast them in a dry frying pan over a medium heat for 4–5 minutes until lightly brown. Keep moving them so they don't burn.
- Double the quantities for four people.

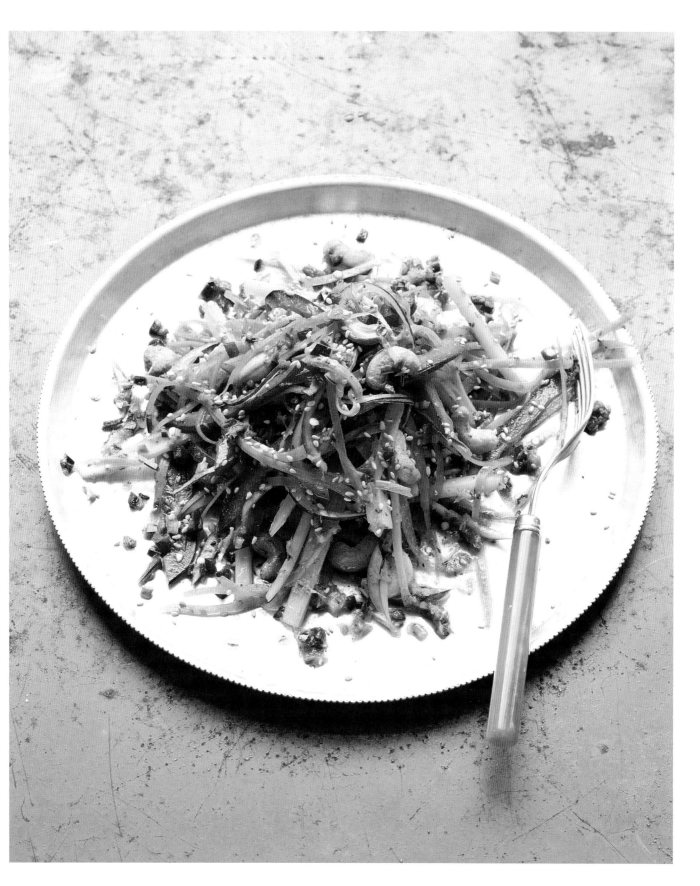

288 KCAL

South Indian Hot and Sour Lentil Soup

Serves 2

Ingredients

2 tbsp olive oil

1 tsp cumin seeds

5–6 fresh curry leaves (optional)

½ onion (red or white), peeled and finely chopped

1 garlic clove, peeled and finely chopped

1cm/½in piece fresh ginger, peeled and finely chopped

1 tbsp South Indian Spice Rub (see p.18)

½ tsp salt

2 tbsp tomato purée (paste)

100g/3½oz/scant ½ cup red lentils, rinsed through in cold water

850ml/1½ pints/3¾ cups low-salt vegetable or chicken stock (broth)

½–1 tsp tamarind paste

a small handful of chopped fresh coriander (cilantro)

This is a delicious, hearty soup that is easy to make with your South Indian Spice Rub, so no need to worry about mixing spices or taking ten jars out of your storecupboard! The spices include health-boosting properties and the tamarind used in this recipe is known for its powerful antioxidant and mineral benefits. The lentils provide a protein burst which keeps you satisfied for a long time; add in garlic and ginger and you are onto a winner in the health and taste stakes!

Method

Heat the olive oil in a medium saucepan over a medium heat. When the oil is hot, throw in the cumin seeds and curry leaves and, as soon as they start to pop, add the onion, garlic and ginger. Cook for 2–3 minutes over a medium heat, so the onion becomes translucent but not brown. Add the spice mix and salt and cook for a further 2–3 minutes. Mix in the tomato purée and stir through for 2 minutes. Add the lentils and stir a few times until they are coated with the onion and tomato mix, then pour in the stock. Bring to the boil, then reduce the heat to low and cook for about 20 minutes. The lentils should be soft and there should be enough soupy liquid (if it is getting thick, add more hot water).

When the lentils are soft, bring to a simmer then swirl through the tamarind paste and cook gently for a further 5 minutes. Garnish with chopped coriander. If you want to make it more sour, add more tamarind.

Tips

• You can make this as hot and as sour as you like. I make it a winter dish by adding more lentils and a lighter summery dish by adding fewer to make it more of a sour and light broth.

• I have used red lentils for this soup, but you can use any variety, just make sure to check the cooking times for other lentils as they can take longer (mung beans or brown lentils work well in this recipe).

• Try adding a couple of handfuls of spinach to the soup for even more goodness. This recipe can be doubled for four people.

Speedy Aromatic Moroccan Chorba with Orzo

140 KCAL

Using your Moroccan spice mix, you can produce so many delicious dishes full of nutritious spices quickly, and this is a speedy vegetarian version of a hearty Moroccan soup. Chorba is a type of Moroccan soup that usually includes vermicielli or small pasta. I have added orzo to this recipe as the texture feels good and the shape of the orzo is very appealing. The spice rub includes so many aromatic spices, such as cumin, citrusy coriander seeds, cinnamon and paprika, all containing vitamins and minerals to support health and digestion. This is a hearty, tasty soup which will not only leave you full but feeling healthy too.

Method

Heat the olive oil in a large pan over a medium heat. When the oil is hot, add the onion and garlic and cook for 2–3 minutes. Add the Moroccan Spice Rub and salt, and stir through for 2 minutes, then add the tomato, tomato purée and celery and chickpeas. Cook over a medium heat for 2 minutes then pour in the vegetable stock. Bring to the boil then reduce the heat to a simmer, cover with a lid and cook for 10 minutes. Add the orzo and parsley and continue cooking for a further 7–10 minutes. Check the seasoning and serve.

Tips

- Use any seasonal vegetables you like.
- A fresh squeeze of lime or lemon when serving the soup adds an extra zing. Double the ingredients for four people.
- Substitute the orzo for any small wholewheat pasta if wished.

Serves 2

Ingredients

1 tbsp olive oil
½ red onion, peeled and finely chopped
1 small garlic clove, peeled and finely chopped
½ tbsp Moroccan Spice Rub (see p.19)
1 medium fresh tomato, roughly chopped
1 tsp tomato purée (paste)
1 celery stalk, diced
85g/3oz½ cup canned chickpeas
1 litre/1¾ pints/4 cups low-salt vegetable stock (broth)
a small handful of orzo (about 15g/½oz)
a small handful of fresh parsley leaves

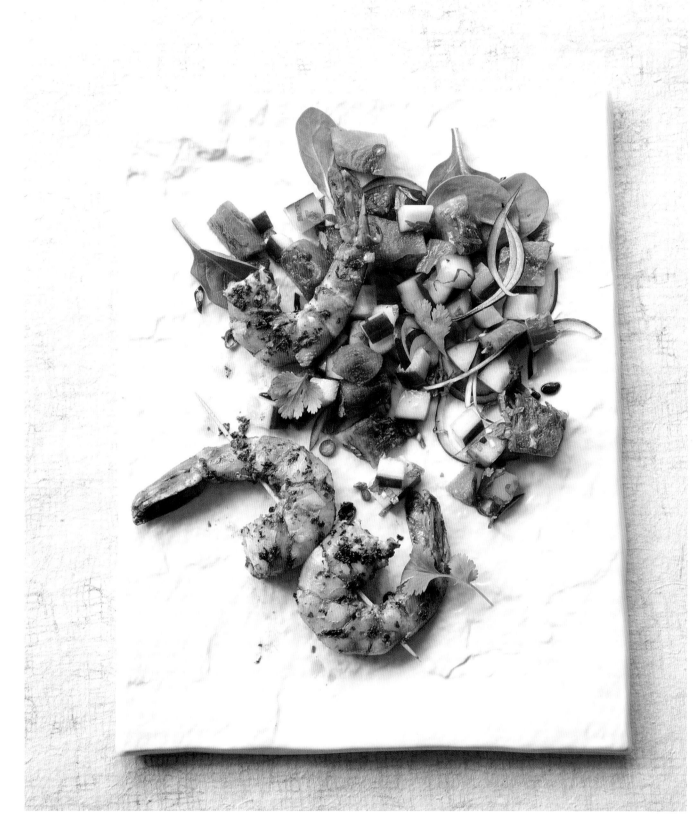

Spicy Prawns with Watermelon Salsa

This tastes like an intricate dish but is very simple to prepare. Luxurious Madagascan prawns coated in flavourful spices and eaten with a cool, ruby-coloured watermelon salsa, this is the dish to make when you want to impress your friends when they come around for a 'quick' lunch. The cumin, chilli and coriander combine to give you triple health benefits and the mint and fresh coriander bring a sweet freshness to the dish.

Method

In a bowl, combine all the ingredients for the marinade and when mixed together, add the prawns. Cover and set aside while you make the salsa.

For the salsa, place the onion, cucumber, chilli and mint in a bowl. Carefully mix in the watermelon and squeeze over the lime juice. Cover and chill in the refrigerator to allow the flavours to meld together.

Preheat the grill to medium.

Thread the prawns onto skewers and grill for 2–3 minutes (depending on the size of the prawns) on each side until cooked.

Scatter the spinach leaves over a large flat plate. Pour over the watermelon salsa, adding the remaining coriander leaves and the salt and pepper on top. Lay the prawn skewers over the salsa and serve with a squeeze of lime.

Tips

- If you can't get Madagascan prawns, use tiger prawns instead.
- This lunch works well for four people by just doubling the ingredients.

Serves 2

You will need 2 small skewers or 1 large skewer (pre-soak if wooden)

Ingredients

8–10 uncooked peeled large prawns (shrimp)
1 small bag (about 75g/2½oz) baby spinach or salad leaves
a squeeze of lime, to garnish

For the marinade

juice of ½ lime
a small handful of fresh coriander (cilantro), finely chopped, save a few leaves for the salsa
¼ tsp salt
1 tsp olive oil
½ tsp ground coriander
½ tsp ground cumin
½ tsp chopped green or red chilli

For the watermelon salsa

½ small red onion, finely sliced
¼ cucumber, peeled and finely diced
¼ medium red chilli, finely chopped
a large handful fresh mint, roughly chopped
175g/6oz diced watermelon
juice of ½ lime
¼ tsp salt
a sprinkling of freshly ground black pepper

323 KCAL

Serves 2

Ingredients

225g/8oz flank steak, sliced into even thin strips
toasted sesame seeds, for sprinkling (optional)
1 tbsp chopped fresh coriander (cilantro) leaves, to garnish

For the marinade

1 tsp Szechuan-Style Spice Rub (see p.19)
1 tbsp soy sauce
2 tbsp Shaoxing wine or dry sherry
1 garlic clove, finely chopped
1cm/½in piece fresh ginger, peeled and chopped or grated
½ tsp sesame oil
salt and freshly ground black pepper
1 tbsp vegetable oil, for cooking

For the courgettini

2 medium courgettes (zucchini)
½ red (bell) pepper
¼ medium cucumber

For the dressing

½ red chilli, finely chopped
2 spring onions (scallions), roughly chopped
2 tbsp lemon oil or combine juice of ½ lemon with 1 tbsp olive oil
¼ tsp sesame oil
salt and freshly ground black pepper

Szechuan Flash-Fried Beef and Citrus Courgettini

A lunch to make you feel like you are treating yourself but not over-indulging! It's light, colourful and full of goodness. The beef slices are marinated quickly in warming spices, which will calm your digestive system and keep your immune system strong. The warming taste of the beef is balanced with a cool salad of courgette, red pepper and cucumber strips simply dressed in lemon oil and chilli.

Method

Place the beef slices in a bowl, add all the marinade ingredients and mix to combine. Cover and leave to marinate for 15–20 minutes.

Thinly slice the courgettes (use a vegetable peeler or spiraliser). Bring a large saucepan of water to the boil, add the courgette strips and blanch for 30 seconds. Using a slotted spoon, lift the strips out and immerse in a large bowl of cold water. Once cool, drain and pat dry with kitchen paper.

Thinly slice the red pepper, then peel the cucumber and cut in half. Spoon out the watery seeds and slice the flesh into strips. In a large bowl, combine the red pepper, courgettes and cucumber.

Mix the dressing ingredients together and pour over the vegetables.

Heat the vegetable oil in a hot frying pan. Shake the marinade off the beef and quickly fry the beef for 1 minute. Don't add too many strips to the pan at a time or the beef may begin to stew. Put each batch of fried beef onto a plate and allow to rest for 2–3 minutes.

Add the beef to the salad, then sprinkle with toasted sesame seeds (if using) and garnish with the chopped coriander leaves.

Tips

- Try chicken breast instead of beef.
- For a vegetarian option, use firm tofu cubes or even paneer cubes.
- You can buy toasted sesame seeds, or I toast them in a dry frying pan over a medium heat for 4–5 minutes until lightly brown. Keep moving them so they don't burn.
- This recipe also works well upscaled for a family for four. Just double the ingredients.

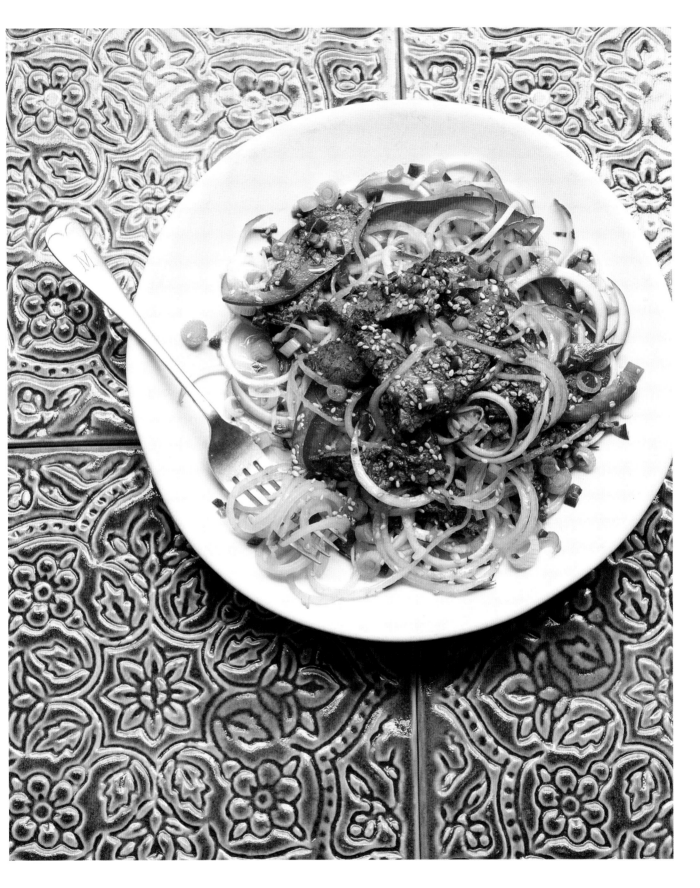

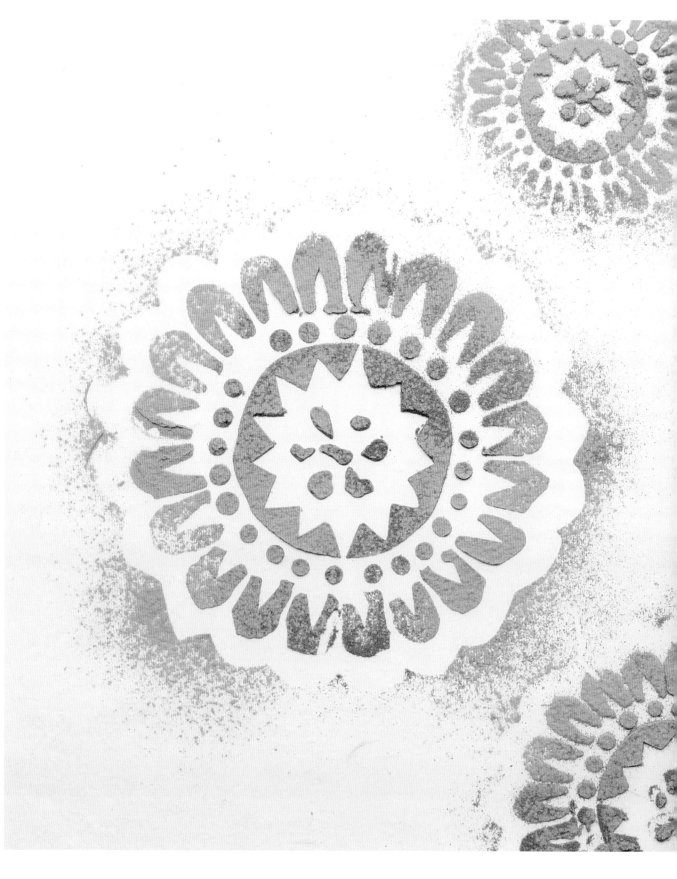

Effortless Dinners

Effortless, tasty and nutritious dishes for dinner that are simple to cook and are healthy, flavourful meals – that's the key to enjoying your evening and to the *Spice Yourself Slim* way of eating.

Most of us lead busy lives with the demands of work, family and a fast-moving world around us, so in the evenings we don't have the time or inclination to spend hours cooking, but we still want to eat well and have meals to enjoy at the end of the day as well as being healthy. My effortless dinners show you how to achieve this. There's so much choice and a variety of flavours and spices and all are low calorie.

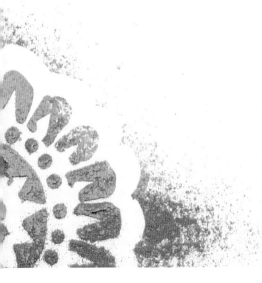

Lively Lagos Fish

Serves 4

Ingredients

500g/1lb 2oz cherry tomatoes,
    scored around the middle
1 large red (bell) pepper,
    deseeded and chopped
    into quarters
3 garlic cloves, peeled and
    roughly chopped
1 red onion, peeled and
    finely chopped
2 habanero chillies, roughly
    chopped, or more if you want
    it extra hot
1 tsp cumin seeds
2 tbsp olive oil
¼ tsp salt
½ tsp grated nutmeg
1 tsp sweet paprika
1 tbsp cider vinegar
4 tilapia fillets

For the stir-fry

1 tbsp groundnut (peanut) oil
2.5cm/1in piece fresh ginger,
    peeled and finely chopped
200g/7oz Tenderstem broccoli
150g/5¼oz spinach or spring
    greens, roughly chopped

Tips

I'm using tilapia here instead of
catfish (it's hard to find a live one!)
but you can use any firm white fish.
Brill would be good. This sauce
also works well with chicken and
meat. I suggest eating this with
stir-fried spring green vegetables.

My first job after leaving university was working for a Nigerian Chief living in London, and we made several trips to Lagos and Oyo for business. Lagos is an amazing city – dusty, busy, noisy and intriguing. The roads are shared equally with cars and people selling books, pots, pans, clothes and, of course, food. My Nigerian colleague Kofi was speeding down one of these busy roads when he screeched to a halt, reversed back, and beckoned to a lady with a bucket on the roadside. After a few minutes, he loaded a wriggling plastic bag on to our back seat and we sped off again. A smiling Kofi told me that we would eat well that evening. The wriggling bag contained an ugly and huge catfish! I was worried about eating it, but Kofi disappeared into the kitchen and reappeared 45 minutes later with a large platter of steaming white fish with a spicy red-hot salsa. It was absolutely delicious. The simple fish was dressed in local spices, a recipe Kofi said came from his mother, his mother's mother and generations before him. A mixture of chillies – habanero for heat and paprika for sweetness – and the spices, cumin and nutmeg that make up this tasty sauce for the fish. It's sweet with a few fiery chillies to move your metabolism and boost your antioxidant and vitamin levels.

Method

Preheat the oven to 220°C/425°F/Gas mark 7. Place the tomatoes, pepper, garlic, onion and chillies in a baking tray. Sprinkle over the cumin seeds, olive oil and salt, and bake in the hot oven for 10–15 minutes until the tomatoes and peppers are slightly charred. Take out of the oven and allow to cool. When cool, peel the skin off the tomatoes and pepper.

Place all the ingredients except the fish in a blender and blend until smooth. Sprinkle the nutmeg over the sauce and mix in the paprika and vinegar, then pour into a pan and warm over a very low heat for 10 minutes. Check the seasoning, adding salt if needed.

Heat the groundnut oil for the stir-fry in a wok. When smoking hot, add the ginger and mix for 1 minute. Quickly add the broccoli and stir-fry for 3 minutes, or until almost soft. Add the spinach or spring greens with a splash of water and a seasoning of salt and pepper.

Cook the fish in a steamer for 4–5 minutes. (Chicken will take longer to steam, about 15–20 minutes.)

Place the vegetable stir-fry on a large plate and arrange the fish on top. Pour on the chilli sauce and serve.

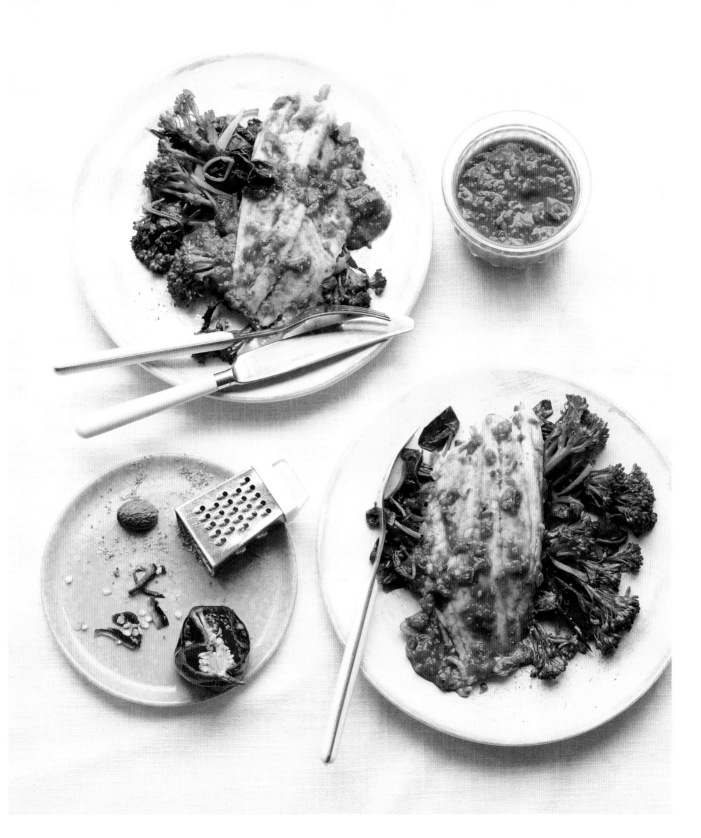

Comforting South Indian Rainbow Vegetables

Serves 4

Ingredients

3 tbsp olive oil

1 tsp fenugreek seeds

5cm/2in piece fresh ginger, peeled and finely chopped

2 tbsp South Indian Spice Rub (see p.18)

½ tsp salt

3 large vine-ripened tomatoes (about 400g/14oz), diced into small cubes

1 tbsp tomato purée (paste)

60ml/2fl oz hot water plus 4 tbsp for the sauce

2 carrots, peeled and cut into discs

½ small cauliflower, cut into very small florets, save some of the good outer leaves

100g/3½oz runner (string) beans, cut into 2.5cm/1in pieces

85g/3oz/¾ cup frozen or fresh garden peas

5 tbsp thick plain yogurt

juice of ½ lemon

a small bunch of fresh coriander (cilantro), roughly chopped

This is a flavourful, hearty main dish, colourful and bursting with healthy spices – cumin, coriander, cloves, fenugreek and turmeric. Fenugreek is a key part of the South Indian Spice Rub. It is one of the oldest plants in the Mediterranean and in Asia and is even mentioned in original Egyptian writings. Fenugreek seeds are thought to be rich in iron, potassium, calcium and many other minerals, so use your South Indian Spice Rub and you will create a fantastic healthy and low-fat meal in no time.

Method

Heat a large saucepan over a medium heat, and when hot, add the olive oil and the fenugreek seeds. Stir for 1 minute in the oil and, as the seeds begin to sizzle, add the ginger, South Indian Spice Rub and the salt. Cook the spices for 1–2 minutes, then add the fresh tomatoes, the tomato purée and 2 tablespoons hot water. Reduce the heat to low and leave for 3–4 minutes, or until the tomatoes have mashed in and the sauce is smooth. If it is catching on the base of the pan, add another tablespoon of water. When the sauce is smooth, add the cauliflower florets and cook for 2 minutes. Add the remaining vegetables and cook for a further 3–4 minutes. Pour in the hot water and bring to the boil. Reduce the heat to a simmer and leave to cook until the vegetables are tender. Turn the heat off and allow to cool.

In a small bowl, whisk the yogurt until smooth then add to the cooled curry. Slowly bring the heat up again and squeeze in the lemon juice. Sprinkle with the coriander leaves and serve.

Tip

You can use any vegetables you like or add chickpeas instead of some of the vegetables, if you prefer.

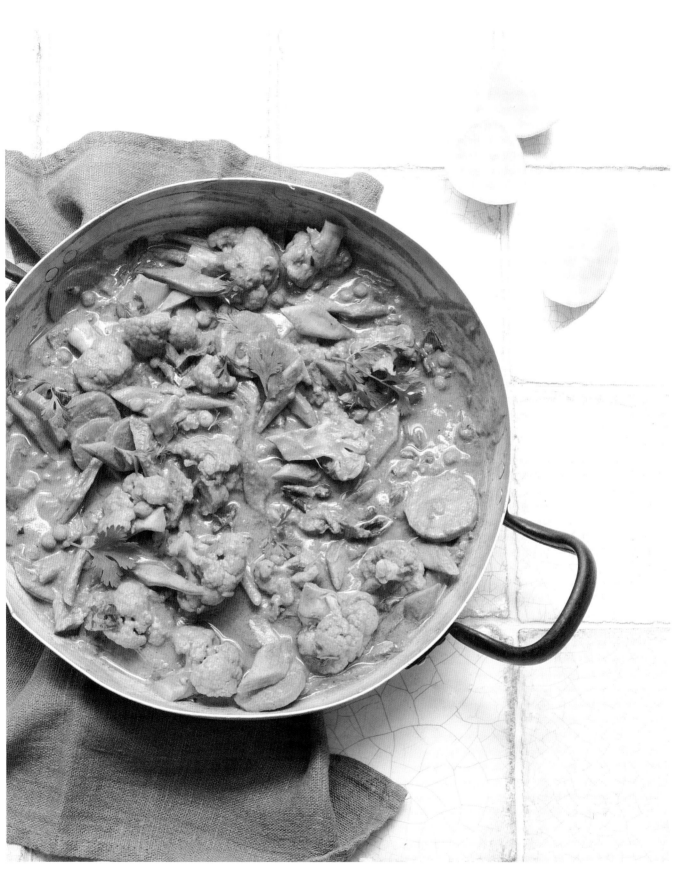

Filling Freekeh Pilaf and Sumac Ricotta

Serves 4

Ingredients

For the freekeh pilav

2 tbsp olive oil
2 garlic cloves, peeled and
   finely chopped
8–10 asparagus spears
½ red (bell) pepper, deseeded
   and chopped into small cubes
a small bunch of kale,
   finely chopped
½ can (118g/4oz) cannellini beans,
   drained
100g/3½oz/scant ½ cup freekeh
1 tsp ground cumin
1 tsp ground cinnamon
2 tbsp harissa
hot low-salt vegetable or
   chicken stock (broth), quantity
   according to the instructions for
   cooking the freekeh
a small handful of fresh flat-leaf
   parsley leaves, chopped
a small handful of fresh coriander
   (cilantro), chopped
zest of ½ lemon (use ½ of the
   lemon used for juicing)
juice of 1 small lemon

For the ricotta

30g/1oz/¼ cup ricotta cheese
1 tsp ground sumac
¼ red onion, peeled and very
   finely sliced
freshly ground black pepper

Eating well to all of us means feeling good and full. Traditional foods filled with spices do make us feel this way. Cumin and cinnamon add layers of warm flavour, which is immensely satisfying as they smell and taste good, while the enticing deep red colour and citrusy taste of sumac is a lovely (and calorie-free) addition to this dish. Freekeh, an ancient grain (mentioned in the Bible), has a nutty, smoky texture and absorbs all the flavours you add to it. It is still commonly used in salads and hot dishes in the Middle East. Freekeh is a grain that's harvested and roasted when young (actually it is 'set on fire' until the outer husk falls off and this gives it its smoky and multi-layered taste). It has been called a 'superfood' because it is high in fibre and protein, with a low glycaemic index (GI) and is rich in calcium, iron and zinc. It is also low in fat.

Method

Heat the oil in a saucepan over a medium heat. Add the garlic, vegetables and beans and cook for 2–3 minutes. Add the freekeh, then stir in the cumin, cinnamon and harissa. Add the stock and bring to the boil. Reduce the heat and simmer for 15–20 minutes or according to the packet instructions until the freekeh is cooked.

Meanwhile, get the ricotta ready. Mix 3 tablespoons lemon juice and sumac powder together in a bowl. Add the red onion, then pour this mixture over the ricotta cheese and mix until the cheese is coated all over. Sprinkle with black pepper and set aside.

When the freekeh is cooked, mix in the herbs and the remaining lemon juice and lemon zest. Serve with ricotta cheese and sumac mixture.

Tips

- Use wholegrain cracked freekeh in this recipe as it will cook quickly. Some varieties require soaking for 15 minutes prior to cooking, so check the packet instructions before using.
- The freekeh pilaf can be eaten hot or cold as a salad.
- Try to find firm ricotta as this will hold the spices better.

Two-Spice Salmon with Magnificent Mango Salsa

This is one of the simplest yet most delicious dishes you can ever make. It's light, citrusy and uses only two storecupboard spices, both packed with flavour and health-boosting properties – cumin is an excellent source of iron and coriander contains high levels of minerals, such as potassium and zinc, and is high in vitamin C. Combined with the salmon, which is full of omega-3 fatty acids (great for your brain and heart), this is a very healthy dish.

The salsa looks magnificent and it tastes great too. The crunchy red pepper, fresh onion, gentle heat of the chilli and the soft sweetness of the mangoes, all topped with aromatic cumin, really work well with the spiciness of the salmon. Make this salsa ahead of the salmon so that the flavours can meld nicely. Eat for either lunch or a light dinner.

Method

Preheat the oven to 200°C/400°F/Gas mark 6.

To make the salsa, in a large bowl, toss the mangoes, mint, red onion, coriander, lime juice, 1 tablespoon olive oil, red pepper and red chilli together then sprinkle with the ground cumin. Cover and set aside.

Combine the fresh coriander and coriander stalks, salt, 2 tablespoons olive oil, green chilli, lime juice and mint leaves in a food processor and pulse for about 15–30 seconds until a rough paste is formed. Keep it rough and moist. I like to pound the mixture in a pestle and mortar but it works by pulsing in a food processor too. Mix in the lime zest, ground coriander and ground cumin. You should have a vibrant green mixture.

Lightly score the top of the fish with a sharp knife. Arrange the fish on a non-stick baking tray then spread a portion of the paste across each fillet. Sprinkle over the remaining olive oil and cover with foil loosely. Place the baking tray in the hottest part of the oven and bake for 6 minutes, then remove the foil and continue cooking for a further 4–6 minutes until the salmon is cooked through. Serve with the salsa.

Serves 4

Ingredients

- a large bunch (about 50g/1¾oz) of fresh coriander (cilantro), roughly chopped, including the stalks
- ½ tsp salt
- 4 tbsp olive oil
- 1 medium red or green chilli, roughly chopped
- 1 fresh lime – zest ½ lime and juice it all
- 10 fresh mint leaves
- 1 tbsp ground coriander
- 1 tbsp ground cumin
- 4 medium salmon fillets

For the magnificent mango salsa

- 2 ripe mangoes, peeled and cut into small cubes
- 10 fresh mint leaves, finely chopped
- ½ medium red onion, peeled and finely chopped
- a small bunch (about 15g/½oz) of fresh coriander (cilantro) leaves, roughly chopped
- 1 tbsp lime juice
- 1 tbsp olive oil
- 1 red (bell) pepper, finely diced
- ½ medium red chilli, finely chopped
- ¼ tsp ground cumin

Roman Holiday Seafood Parcels

Serves 4

Ingredients

2 tbsp olive oil

zest and juice of ½ lemon

1½ tbsp Mediterranean Spice Rub (see p.19)

2 garlic cloves, peeled and finely chopped

100g/3½oz peeled raw prawns (shrimp)

150g/5¼oz squid rings

100g/3½oz skinned salmon, cut into 7.5cm/3in pieces

250g/9oz cod loin or white fish, cut into 7.5cm/3in pieces

½ tsp fennel seeds

½ tsp salt

10–12 grinds of black pepper

100ml/3½fl oz/scant ½ cup low-salt fish or chicken stock (broth)

1 tbsp tomato purée (paste)

150g/5¼oz small vine tomatoes, sliced

8 fresh thyme or lemon thyme sprigs

The first time I went to Rome, I stumbled across a wonderful small restaurant down a narrow back street. I always wait to see what the locals are ordering and eating before I make my choice. At this charming place I found that the locals were tucking into a foil paper parcel but I couldn't see what was in it. All I could smell was the deep, chilli and herb aroma coming from these parcels. They were eating a dish of beautiful fresh seafood and fish. I have tried to recreate this, as it was so delicious, simple and healthy. Using my Mediterranean Spice Rub with dried oregano, thyme, dried garlic, chilli and paprika, this makes a healthy and delicious dinner. I have also added fennel seeds, which are high in antioxidants and minerals and calm digestion.

Method

Preheat the oven to 200°C/400°F/Gas mark 6.

Mix the olive oil, lemon juice, lemon zest, Mediterranean Spice Rub and garlic together in a large bowl. Put the seafood and fish into the bowl, sprinkle over the fennel seeds, season with the salt and pepper, and mix again. Set aside for 5 minutes.

Make the fish stock then mix the tomato purée into the hot stock.

Prepare 4 foil parcels on a baking tray and lay equal amounts of tomato slices in each. Divide the fish only (not the seafood yet) between the parcels and pour over an equal amount of the fish stock. Lay 2 thyme sprigs over each parcel, then close each parcel and cook in the hot oven for about 7–10 minutes until the fish is almost cooked. Take out of the oven, carefully add the seafood to the parcels, re-close and return the parcels to the oven for about 5 minutes until everything is cooked.

Serve as a foil parcel with steamed broccoli.

Tip

You can use any firm fish and any seafood including clams, mussels, langoustines (for a dinner party) and crab claws, if you like.

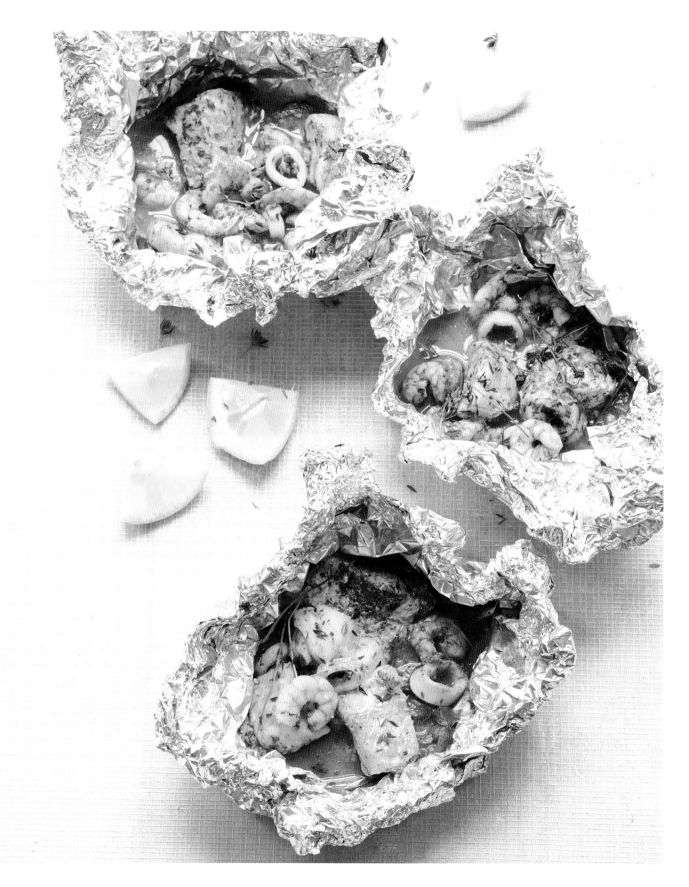

Easy and Lite Saucy Tandoori Chicken

This is the dish we crave when we want an Indian takeaway, but it's normally full of fat and cream and the spices are buried in heavy sauce! In this version, you will taste all the spices – turmeric, Kashmiri chillies, coriander, cloves and cinnamon. Plain yogurt gives the dish a light creamy and healthy taste. It's quick and easy if you use the pre-prepared Tandoori Spice Rub. You can make this for a dinner for the family or make it 'special' for guests by garnishing with thinly sliced roasted almonds and fresh pomegranate seeds.

Serves 4

Ingredients

150g/5¼oz oz/⅔ cup whole plain yogurt
3 tbsp Tandoori Spice Rub (p.18)
1 tsp salt
juice of ½ lemon, keep a dash for squeezing before serving
2 garlic cloves, peeled and finely chopped
5cm/2in piece fresh ginger, peeled and finely chopped
3 tbsp olive oil – 1 tbsp for marinade, 2 tbsp for cooking
4 medium pieces of chicken breast, skinned (if you can get it on the bone, this will be better) and cut into 5cm/2in chunks
1 large onion, peeled and thinly sliced lengthways
1 large beef tomato, chopped into small cubes
2 tbsp tomato purée (paste)
200ml/7fl oz/1 cup hot water
1 small bag (100g/3½oz) baby spinach leaves
a small bunch of fresh coriander (cilantro) leaves, chopped

Method

Using a hand whisk, whisk the yogurt in a bowl until it is smooth, with no lumps and of 'pouring' consistency. This will help the yogurt not separate when cooking. Add 2 tablespoons of the Spice Rub, the salt, lemon juice, garlic, ginger and 1 tablespoon olive oil to the yogurt. Drop in the chicken pieces and mix in well. Cover and leave in the refrigerator to marinate for at least 1 hour, or overnight, to allow the spices to meld together.

When you are ready to cook, preheat the grill as hot as it will go.

Shake the excess marinade off each piece of chicken (keep the marinade for the sauce) and grill for 5 minutes on each side. The chicken should be parcooked and have a slightly charred colour. Set the chicken aside.

To make the sauce, heat a wok or large pan over a medium heat and add the olive oil. When the oil is hot, add the onions and cook until they are soft but not brown. Mix in the remaining Tandoori Spice Rub and cook for 2–3 minutes. Add the tomatoes and tomato purée and cook over a medium heat for a further 3–4 minutes. Add 1 tablespoon water, then turn off the heat and allow to cool.

Whisk the remaining marinade to make it smooth. When the sauce is cool, turn on the heat again to very low and slowly pour in the marinade. Cook gently for 5 minutes, then fold in the chicken pieces. Turn them a few times to coat in the sauce then pour in the water. Bring to a slow boil then reduce the heat to a simmer, partially cover with a lid, and continue cooking until you have a medium sauce, about 8–10 minutes.

Mix in the spinach leaves and, as they wilt, sprinkle over the coriander and a big squeeze of lemon juice.

Tips

• You can substitute fish for the chicken. Salmon and tilapia go well, as do prawns, and a mix of vegetables also works well.
• Eat your tandoori meal with a green salad or cauliflower rice.

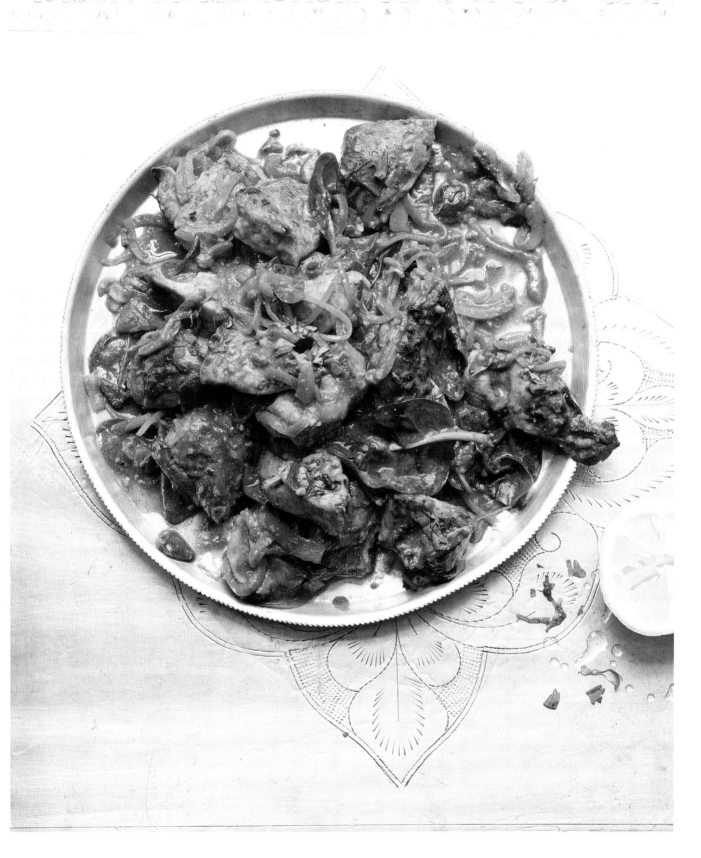

Gobi Muttar (Golden Crumbed Cauliflower and Peas)

Serves 4

Ingredients

1 medium cauliflower
3 tbsp olive oil
5cm/2in piece fresh ginger, peeled and finely chopped
1 tbsp ground turmeric
½ tsp hot red chilli powder
1 green chilli, finely chopped
½ tsp salt
1 tbsp ground coriander, plus ½ tsp for the garnish
300g/10½oz canned peeled cherry tomatoes (including the tomato juice)
a large handful of fresh coriander (cilantro), stems and leaves chopped separately
100g/3½oz/scant 1 cup petit pois
juice of ½ lime

This is a family favourite and a speciality of my mum's. She calls this a softer, lighter version of the traditional Gobi Aloo (cauliflower and potatoes) dish. Cauliflower and spices work so well together, and I think transform this everyday vegetable into a tasty special one. Turmeric is the key spice in this dish. It gives a lovely golden colour but it also adds a health-giving boost. It is a powerful anti-inflammatory, anti-viral and great for fighting infections. Ground coriander is also an anti-inflammatory and is thought to help control blood sugar levels, and chilli will help kick-start your metabolism. At home we eat this with wholewheat chapattis and Cucumber and Mint Raita (see p.143).

Method

To prepare the cauliflower, remove the outer thicker leaves of the cauliflower and discard. Reserve the more tender, greener leaves as they can be added when cooking the florets. Cut the florets off the cauliflower and separate them into small florets. Chop the middle of the cauliflower stem into very small cubes (discard the hard bottom bit) and rinse in cold water.

Heat a large wok over a medium heat and add the olive oil. When the oil is hot, add the ginger and cook for 1 minute. Add the turmeric, chilli powder, green chilli, salt and ground coriander and mix in the hot oil for 2 minutes. Add the tomatoes and fresh coriander stems and cook for 3–4 minutes. When the oil runs to the top, add the cauliflower and cook for 10–12 minutes over a medium heat. If it is sticking at any point, add 1 tablespoon of warm water. When the cauliflower is almost soft, add the petit pois. Reduce the heat to medium-low, cover with a lid and cook for a further 3–4 minutes. Squeeze the lime juice over and sprinkle with coriander leaves to serve.

Tips

- You can use this recipe for different vegetables, such as small diced carrots and green peppers.
- If you can't find petit pois, then use garden peas instead.

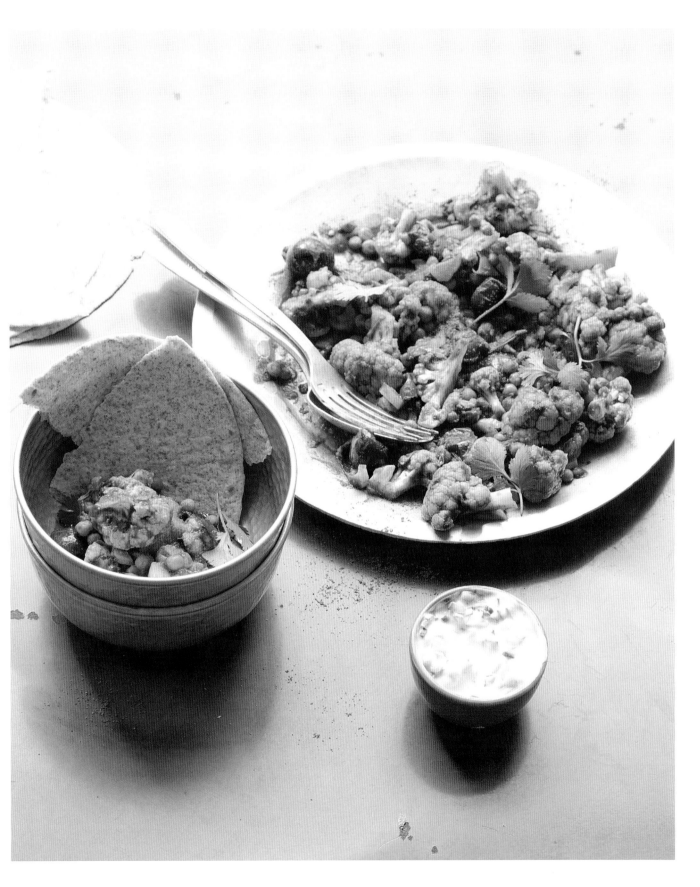

247
KCAL

Mediterranean Stuffed Aubergines

Serves 4

Ingredients

2 large aubergines (eggplants)
3 tbsp olive oil
1 tsp cumin seeds
1 red onion, peeled and
   finely chopped
2 garlic cloves, peeled and
   finely chopped
½ small red chilli, finely chopped
   (optional)
2 tbsp Mediterranean Spice Rub
   (see p.19)
1 tsp salt
freshly ground black pepper
8–10 sunkissed tomatoes,
   roughly chopped
a large handful of fresh
   basil leaves
70g/2½oz/scant ½ cup black
   pitted Kalamata olives
120g/4½oz Greek feta cheese,
   cut into small cubes

Tips

• Add cubed courgettes or red
  peppers if you would like to vary
  the taste.
• If you can't find sunkissed
  tomatoes, then use sun-dried
  ones and if they are in oil,
  shake the oil off before adding
  to the dish.

I believe in having colourful foods on the plate and I love the beautiful dark gloss of an aubergine, which looks like it has been coloured dark by the hot rays of the sun. Unfortunately, although aubergines are good for you, they do need help in terms of taste. Spices really help to introduce flavour to the soft flesh. To give this dish a Mediterranean flavour, just mix in your Mediterranean Spice Rub (oregano, thyme combined with chilli flakes, red paprika and dried garlic). I have also added rich aromatic cumin and fresh garlic. These will aid digestion and the garlic is full of vitamin C, manganese and vitamin B6 and also works hard to keep illnesses at bay as it can strengthen the immune system. This quick and easy dinner is great eaten with with my Cool, Healthy Spinach Yogurt (see p.143).

Method

Preheat the oven to 180°C/350°F/Gas mark 4.

Cut each aubergine in half lengthways. Score the aubergine flesh with some deep cuts a few times but don't cut all the way through the aubergines.

Place the aubergines on a baking tray and drizzle with 1 tablespoon olive oil. Bake in the hot oven for 12–15 minutes until almost soft. Leave the oven on. Allow the aubergines to cool then scoop out the flesh.

Heat a frying pan over a medium heat and add the remaining olive oil. When the oil is hot, add the cumin seeds and, as soon as they start to sizzle, add the onion, garlic and chilli and cook for 4–5 minutes, or until the onion is soft. Sprinkle in the Mediterranean Spice Rub and mix in the aubergine flesh. Season with salt and pepper and sauté over a high heat for 3–4 minutes. Add the tomatoes and basil leaves, mix, then take the pan off the heat and fold in the olives and feta.

Divide the mixture between the aubergine skins and return to the oven for 10–15 minutes until the stuffing and the skins are cooked.

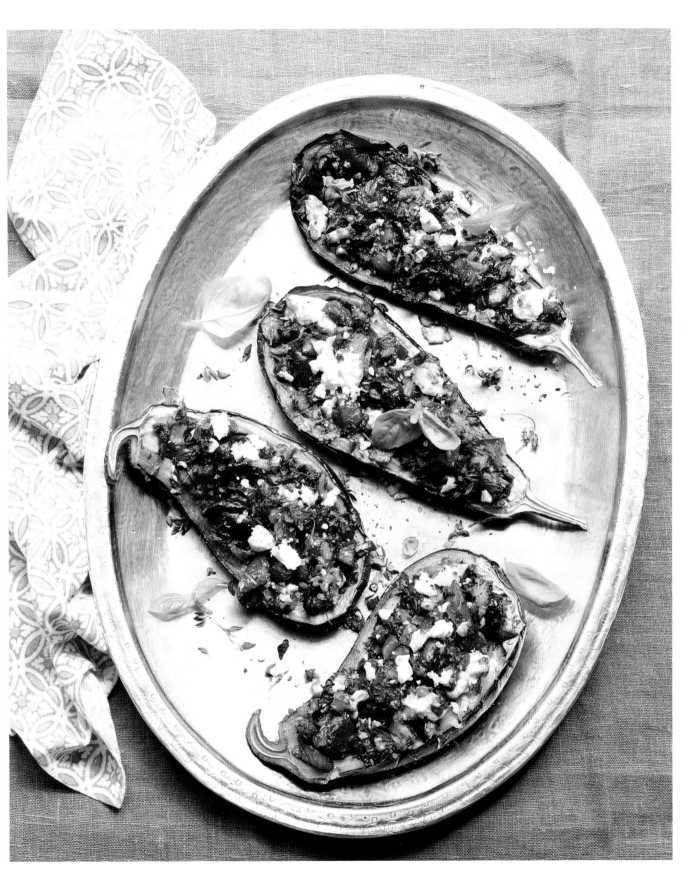

218 KCAL

Quick Treat
Mexican Red Rice

Serves 4

Ingredients

2 tbsp olive oil
2 garlic cloves, peeled and
   finely chopped
1 small onion, peeled and
   finely chopped
¼ tsp salt
1 tsp ground cumin
½ medium jalapeño chilli or
   red mild chilli
½ red or green (bell) pepper
200g/7oz canned black beans
200g/7oz can chopped tomatoes
115g/4oz/½ cup basmati rice,
   washed and drained
300ml/10½fl oz/1¼ cups low-salt
   chicken or vegetable stock
   (broth)
a large handful of fresh coriander
   (cilantro), roughly chopped
juice of ½ lime

Mexican rice is fun and quick to make. It is appetising as it is a lovely red colour and basmati rice has a low glycaemic index (GI) so it makes you feel full for longer. The addition of cumin and garlic soothes your digestion as you eat it.

Method

Heat the oil in a large saucepan over a medium heat. Add the garlic and, as soon as it sizzles, add the onion and cook for 3–4 minutes, or until soft but not brown. Add the salt, cumin, jalapeño chilli, green pepper and the black beans and mix well. Cook for 2 minutes, then add the tomatoes and cook for 3–4 minutes until the tomatoes are mashed in and the mixture is quite dry. Fold in the rice and mix thoroughly until the rice is coated in the tomatoes. Pour in the stock and bring to the boil. Boil for 2 minutes over a medium-high heat then reduce the heat to a simmer. Cover with a tight-fitting lid and leave until all the water has evaporated and the rice is cooked, about 10 minutes.

Stir in the chopped coriander and lime juice and serve.

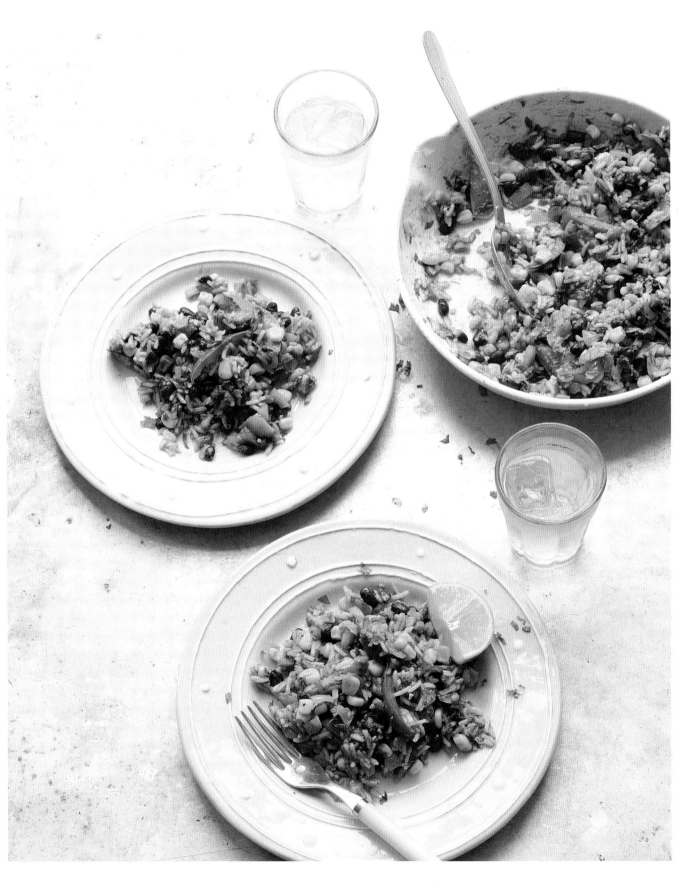

214
KCAL

Sustaining Mexican Black Beans and Peppers

Serves 4

Ingredients

3 tbsp olive oil

3 garlic cloves, peeled and crushed

1 large onion, peeled and roughly chopped

3 tbsp Mexican Spice Rub (p.18)

½ tsp salt

½ tsp chilli (red pepper) flakes

2 x 400g/14oz cans black beans, drained and rinsed

700ml/1¼ pints/3 cups hot water

1 large green (bell) pepper, deseeded and diced

a large handful of fresh coriander (cilantro), finely chopped

Black beans are high in protein, fibre, antioxidants, and iron, so it's no wonder that they have been a staple part of the Mexican diet for over 7,000 years. Combine these health benefits with good spices in your Mexican Spice Rub (smoky chipotle chillies, coriander, cumin, paprika and oregano – all spices rooted in Mexican cuisine) and you have a wholly satisfying and nutritious meal. Cook these beans slowly to bring the flavours together then eat this dish with Papaya and Kiwi Relish (see p.52).

Method

Heat the olive oil in a large saucepan over a medium heat. Add the garlic and, when the garlic begins to sizzle, add the onions and cook for 4–5 minutes, or until they are translucent. Mix in the Mexican Spice Rub, salt and chilli flakes and cook for 2–3 minutes.

Add the black beans and turn a few times until they are coated in the spices. Pour in the water and bring to the boil. Reduce the heat and simmer for 15 minutes.

Add the diced green pepper and simmer for a further 15 minutes. The sauce should be thick. If it is drying out, add more hot water and heat through. Sprinkle the chopped coriander on top and serve with Papaya and Kiwi Relish (see p.52).

Tip

If you can't get black beans, use pinto or kidney beans instead.

Mediterranean Sumac Roast Vegetables with Butter Beans

239 KCAL

This is a quick and easy one-tray satisfying and filling meal. We all know that we need to eat more vegetables but sometimes we just want something tasty! Well, this dish gives you heaps of taste and you can use any vegetables you fancy. Really make your vegetables sing by roasting them with your Mediterranean Spice Rub (an intoxicating mix of aromatic thyme, oregano, chilli flakes and paprika). I have also added sumac, whole carom seeds and garlic cloves. The sumac adds a lively tang and the carom seeds a gentle heat. Carom seeds are known to benefit digestion and ease any tummy bloating. The beans add the necessary protein to complete the meal.

Method

Preheat the oven to 180°C/350°F/Gas mark 4.

Heat the oil in an oven tray or large flat casserole dish over a medium heat. When the oil is hot, throw in the carom seeds and garlic cloves and, as soon as the seeds start to sizzle, quickly add the onions, sweet potatoes, peppers and courgettes. Sprinkle with the salt, Mediterranean Spice Rub and sumac powder, and mix everything together so the vegetables are coated with the herbs and spices.

Place the tray or dish in the hot oven and cook for 10 minutes. Stir in the butter beans, tomatoes and asparagus spears and continue to cook in the oven for a further 10–12 minutes, or until all the vegetables are cooked.

Eat with a green salad.

Serves 4

Ingredients

- 4 tbsp olive oil
- 2 tsp carom seeds
- 2 large garlic cloves, peeled and kept whole but lightly squashed
- 2 red onions, peeled and cut into quarters
- 1 large sweet potato, chopped into small cubes
- 1 large red (bell) pepper, cut into 5cm/2in chunks
- 2 courgettes (zucchini), cut into large chunks
- ½ tsp sea salt
- 2 tbsp Mediterranean Spice Rub (see p.19)
- 1 tbsp ground sumac
- 400g/14oz can butter (lima) beans, drained and rinsed
- 12–15 cherry tomatoes, sliced in half
- 100g/3½oz asparagus spears, woody ends trimmed

Singapore Satay Sticks with Red and White Mooli Slaw

Serves 4

Ingredients

4 large skinless, boneless chicken breasts, cut in 2.5cm/1in cubes

For the marinade

2 garlic cloves, peeled and roughly chopped
2 large shallots, peeled and roughly chopped
2 lemongrass stalks, outer layers peeled and roughly chopped
½ red chilli, roughly chopped
2 tbsp groundnut (peanut) or sunflower oil
juice of 1 lime
1 tsp ground coriander
1 tsp ground turmeric
½ tsp salt
1 tsp soy sauce

For the mooli slaw

1 mooli (daikon), peeled and grated
¼ tsp salt
¼ red onion, thinly sliced
½ tsp grated fresh ginger
100g/3½oz radishes, thinly sliced
1 carrot, cut into julienne
½ red chilli, finely sliced
juice of ½ lime
½ tsp palm sugar
15g/½oz fresh coriander (cilantro) leaves, roughly chopped

The first time I went to Singapore, I was 18 years old and it was a huge eye-opener for me. The first night, we went to a night street food market and ate our way through so much flavourful food, freshly cooked in hot woks and coal barbecues, and this was the first time I ever had satay. I loved that satay was being cooked on almost every street corner and you could just ask for three, four or five sticks and eat it piping hot. Satay is usually simply marinated with turmeric, coriander and lime. Turmeric is a great anti-inflammatory and I believe it can really fuel your brain, so I add it to many of my dishes.

I serve this dish with a refreshing crunchy mooli slaw rather than the more usual peanut sauce. This salad also goes well with other dishes. You can normally buy mooli from Asian and Chinese grocery stores. It is a long white vegetable and has a similar taste to red radishes but is a bit more peppery (I liken it to a mild horseradish taste).

Method

For the marinade, place the garlic, shallots, lemongrass, chilli, groundnut oil and lime juice in a food processor and grind until a thick paste forms. Put the paste in a bowl and add the chicken pieces. Sprinkle over the coriander, turmeric, salt and soy sauce and mix thoroughly. Cover and marinate in the refrigerator for at least 1 hour.

Meanwhile, make the slaw. Place the mooli and the salt in a bowl and leave for 10 minutes. This will remove any of the bitterness from the salad, then drain off any excess water. Add the mooli to the onion, ginger, radish, carrots and chilli in another bowl. Mix the lime juice with the palm sugar and pour over all the ingredients in the bowl. Cover and set aside for 20–30 minutes, then garnish with the coriander leaves.

Presoak 4 long bamboo skewers or 8 small skewers in a bowl of water for 10 minutes. Thread the chicken pieces onto the skewers, pushing them tightly together. Set the marinade aside.

Preheat a grill or barbecue and, when hot, place the skewers under the grill or on the barbecue. Cook for 5 minutes each side, turning halfway through and basting with the marinade until the chicken is a golden colour and cooked through. Serve with the mooli slaw.

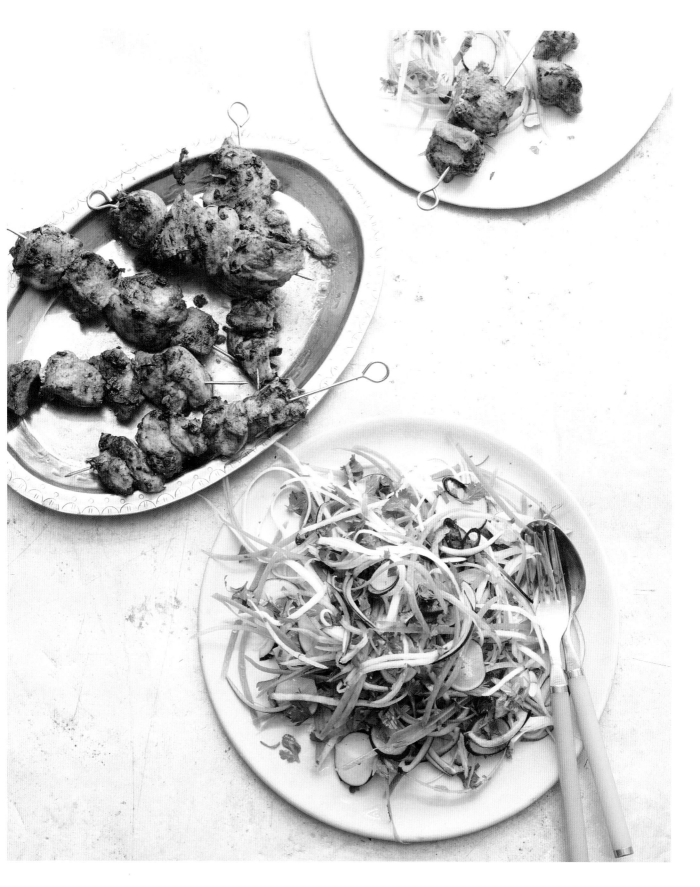

443 KCAL

Slow-Cooked Hanoi Hot Pot

This slow-cooked, sweet, sticky beef dish with spices immediately reminds me of the restaurant where we ate this delicious hotpot in Hanoi. Much of Vietnamese food is quickly prepared, but this dish came in a slow-cook claypot and the depth of flavour was a testament not only to the lovely spices but also to the amount of time it had taken to cook it. Vietnamese food is rightly in vogue because it is very simple and full of locally grown fresh ingredients. Vietnam's climate produces many spices and the Vietnamese have a long tradition of using them in their food for taste but also for their healing powers. This hotpot includes signature spices of star anise and cinnamon with garlic and ginger all producing an intense flavour. Ginger is an anti-inflammatory and aids digestion; garlic is rich in antioxidants; star anise is an antibacterial and super-spice cinnamon will keep glucose levels stable, so not bad for one dinner dish.

Serves 4

Ingredients

500g/1lb 2oz lean braising beef
2 tbsp olive oil
3 large eschalion shallots, peeled and roughly chopped
1 cinnamon stick
2 star anise
2 bay leaves
750ml/1¼ pints/3 cups hot low-salt beef stock (broth)
120g/4½oz shiitake mushrooms (fresh or dried)
3 large carrots, peeled and sliced

For the marinade

2 tbsp dark soy sauce
5cm/2in piece fresh ginger, peeled
2 garlic cloves, peeled
2 hot green chillies, slit down the middle, but don't go all the way through
1 tbsp runny honey

Method

Preheat the oven to 160°C/325°F/Gas mark 3.

Put the beef in a large bowl and add the soy sauce.

Place the ginger, garlic and chilli in a small food processor and chop finely. Add this mixture to the beef. Drizzle in the honey and mix thoroughly. Cover and leave for 10–15 minutes.

Heat the olive oil in an ovenproof heavy-based saucepan over a medium heat. Shake the marinade off the beef (keep the marinade aside) and quickly brown the beef in batches in the oil. Return the meat to the pan and add the shallots, cinnamon stick, star anise and bay leaf. Pour in the marinade and beef stock, then bring to the boil. Place the pan in the hot oven and cook for 1 hour.

After 1 hour, add the shiitake mushrooms and carrots to the beef and cook for a further 45 minutes–1 hour, or until the meat is tender. The sauce should be rich and thick. Check the seasoning and add salt if needed.

Remove the star anise and cinnamon stick before serving with steamed broccoli and kale.

Tip

You can use lean lamb or chicken thighs, if you like.

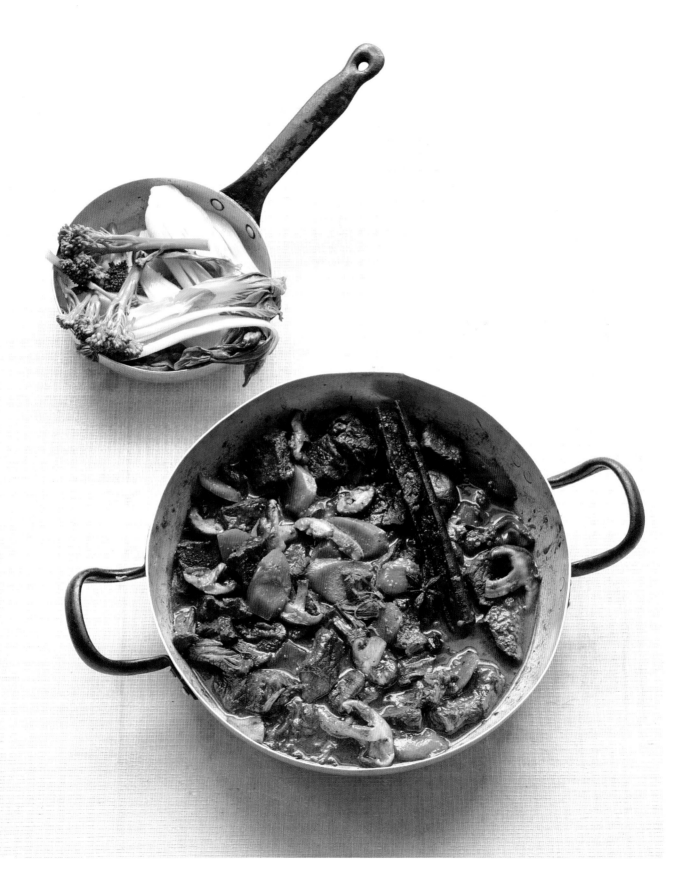

Rajma Masala (Magic Kidney Beans)

I call this a 'magic' dish for two reasons. First, because the flavourful spices here elevate the humble kidney bean into a wonderful dish, and secondly and more importantly, because this is my eldest sister's recipe and she was renowned as having a magic touch when cooking. When Mohinder cooked, we would all wait impatiently and we all tried to copy her – writing down recipes faithfully and being coached, but we never had her touch. She is no longer with us, but her son has given me this recipe. It is a traditional dish cooked in all Punjabi homes, but it is her personal take on it that gives this a special taste. Protein-filled kidney beans are slow-cooked together with cumin, garlic, ginger and chilli. These spices add flavour but also help to calm the digestion as kidney beans can be heavy on the stomach.

Serves 4

Ingredients

2 x 400g/14oz kidney beans,
    do not drain
2 tsp cumin seeds
25g/1oz butter
1 tbsp olive oil
2½cm/1in piece fresh ginger,
    peeled and grated
1 tsp ground turmeric
1 tsp garam masala
2 small green chillies,
    finely chopped
1 large onion, finely chopped
½ can (200g/7oz) chopped plum
    tomatoes and juice
1 tsp salt
a small handful of fresh coriander
    (cilantro) leaves

For the easy spiced cauliflower rice

1 small cauliflower, leaves
    removed
½ tbsp cumin seeds
1 tsp olive oil
¼ tsp salt
a small handful of fresh coriander
    (cilantro), stems and leaves
    separated

Tip

I am using canned kidney beans as they are quick and easy but you can use any bean you like – borlotti and black-eyed peas also work well.

Method

Pour the beans and the water from the cans into a bowl then sprinkle 1 teaspoon cumin seeds over the top. Cover and set aside for 1–2 hours.

Heat the butter and olive oil in a large pan over a medium heat. Add the remaining cumin seeds and cook for 1 minute. Add the ginger, turmeric, garam masala and green chillies, and stir in the heat for a further minute. Add the onion and cook for about 3–4 minutes until it is soft and almost brown. Add the tomatoes and juice and cook over a low-medium heat for 4–5 minutes until the tomatoes are mashed in.

Strain the kidney beans but reserve the water. Add the beans to the pan with the onions and tomatoes and cook for 2 minutes. Season with the salt then pour in the reserved water. Bring to the boil then reduce the heat and simmer for 30–40 minutes, or until the kidney beans should still hold their shape but the texture should be creamy.

Meanwhile, to make the cauliflower rice, grate the cauliflower on a grater, or you can pulse the cauliflower in a food processor. Heat the oil in a pan over a medium heat. Add the cumin seeds and, as soon as the seeds start to sizzle, about 2 minutes, add the cauliflower and coriander stems. Reduce the heat and lightly sauté for 5–7 minutes. Sprinkle with the salt and coriander leaves.

Sprinkle the coriander leaves over the kidney beans and serve with the cauliflower rice.

Mum's Curcumin Loaded Chana Daal

This is my mum's recipe – chana daal is a 'meaty' daal with a wonderful texture which we would look forward to eating as a family. It is a traditional North Indian dish and provides vitamins, protein and iron. Importantly, this dish provides a double hit of turmeric as it is added to the daal when boiling and to the sauce. Turmeric is a true power spice packed with antioxidants and helping to ease inflammation. Every day new research findings are showing the positive health effects of turmeric. This recipe also includes chilli, ground coriander and cumin – all wonderful health-giving spices, so each mouthful will not only taste delightful but also fuel you with goodness.

This daal can be either eaten as a one-bowl dinner or as a soup. It tastes even better the next day so make double the quantity.

Method

Rinse the daal so the water runs clear, then soak in a bowl of cold water for at least 2 hours, or overnight.

Bring the water to the boil in a large saucepan. When the water starts to boil, add the daal and 1 teaspoon ground turmeric. Partially cover the pan and cook over a medium-high heat for 30 minutes. The water may need skimming. After 30 minutes, turn up the heat to high and cook for a further 10–15 minutes until the daal is soft and the water is absorbed into the daal. The daal should retain its shape but still be soft.

Heat the oil in a deep frying pan over a medium heat. Add the cumin seeds and, as soon as they start to they sizzle, add the garlic and ginger. Mix for 1 minute then add the chopped onion, coriander stems and green chilli and cook for 4–5 minutes until the onion is soft and almost brown. Add the spices – the remaining turmeric, the ground coriander, chilli powder and the salt – and stir through for 1–2 minutes. Add the canned tomatoes and juice and the tomato purée, then add the warm water and leave to meld together for about 8–10 minutes over a low-medium heat until the tomatoes are mashed down and the sauce is thick. At this stage, add the spinach leaves and cook for 1–2 minutes until wilted.

When the daal is soft, spoon the sauce into the daal and simmer for 5–10 minutes. The daal will thicken. Mix in the coriander leaves and serve.

Serves 4

Ingredients

200g/7oz dried chana daal
2 litres/3½ pints cold water
2 tsp ground turmeric

For the sauce

2 tbsp olive oil
1 tsp cumin seeds
2 garlic cloves, finely chopped
5cm/2in piece fresh ginger, peeled and grated
1 medium onion, finely chopped
28g/1oz fresh coriander (cilantro), stems and leaves chopped separately
1 green chilli, finely chopped
1 tsp ground coriander
½ tsp chilli powder
¾ tsp salt
200g/7oz canned chopped tomatoes
1 tbsp tomato purée (paste)
4–5 tbsp warm water
160g/5½oz young spinach leaves, roughly chopped

Tips

- Do not get chana daal mixed up with split pea lentils – they are different types of lentils. You can use any lentil for this recipe but adjust cooking time accordingly.
- If you want to make the sauce quicker, you can omit the onions.
- Serve with wholemeal pitta bread.

213
KCAL

Sticky Adobo Spiced Grilled Pork Chops

Adobo is a seasoning that was historically used to preserve meat – a delicious mixture of garlic, oregano, paprika, turmeric, cumin and vinegar (the spices can vary from country to country). It is now widely used in Spanish, Caribbean and Philippine kitchens as a marinade, as it is a delightful mix and works well with fish and all meats.

I am using ancho chillies in this recipe. These chillies are dried, smoked, Mexican chillies. They have a sweet, smoky flavour and add real depth to this marinade. The fusions of these chillies and spices give these pork chops a real taste boost, and the spices have many health properties.

Serves 4

Ingredients

2 medium pork chops, trimmed and any fat removed

For the adobo marinade

3 small ancho chillies, finely chopped or 1 tsp chilli (red pepper) flakes
½ tbsp ground paprika
½ tbsp ground cumin
1 tsp ground turmeric
2 garlic cloves, peeled and finely chopped
1 tsp dried oregano
1 tbsp apple cider vinegar
3 tbsp freshly squeezed orange juice
2 tbsp runny honey
2 tbsp olive oil
½ tsp salt, or to taste

Method

Combine all the ingredients for the adobo marinade in a bowl. Add the pork chops and mix well, making sure each pork chop is coated with the marinade. Cover and allow to marinate in the refrigerator for 2 hours, or overnight.

Preheat the grill to high.

Shake the marinade off the pork chops and set aside to use as a baste when grilling the meat. Place the pork chops on the wire rack in the grill pan and cook under the grill for 5–6 minutes on each side, or until cooked through, basting regularly with the marinade. Make sure the meat is cooked through and not pink. Slice the chops thinly and serve with Shaved Fennel, Fennel Seeds, Cucumber and Pomegranate Side Salad (see p.138).

Tips

- If you can't get ancho chillies, use dried chilli flakes or Kashmiri chillies.
- This works really well with chicken too.

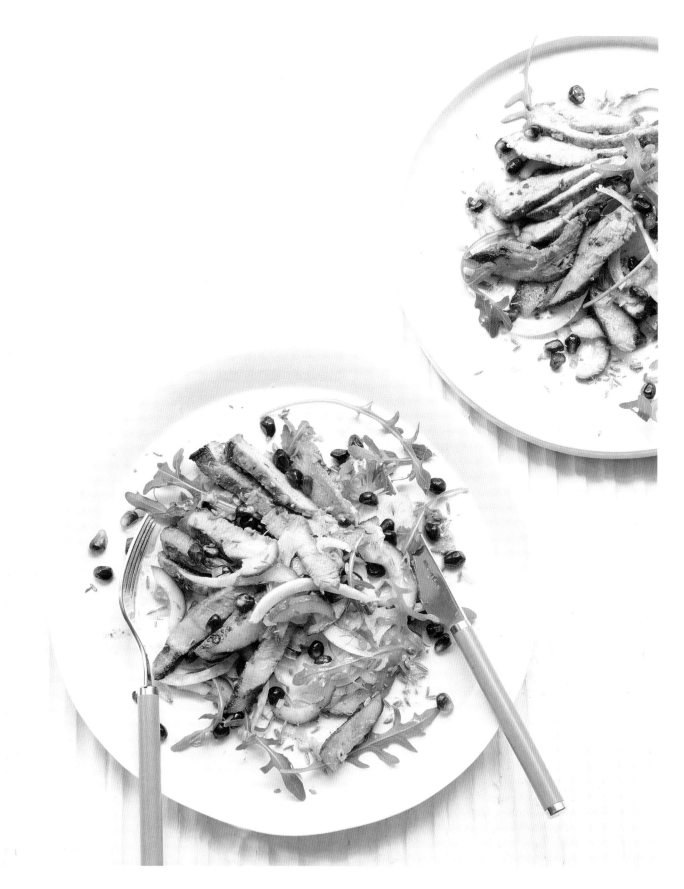

Versatile Monkfish Chermoula

Serves 4

Ingredients

300g/10½oz monkfish fillets, cut into thick 10–15cm/ 4–6in chunks

For the chermoula marinade

1 tbsp cumin seeds
1 tbsp coriander seeds
½ tsp ground paprika
1 tsp chilli (red pepper) flakes or cayenne pepper (optional)
½ tsp finely chopped fresh ginger
1 garlic clove, peeled and finely chopped
5–6 saffron threads, soaked in 2 tbsp warm water for 3–4 minutes
juice of 1 lemon, set aside 1 tbsp for the fish
2 tbsp olive oil
½ tsp salt
a large handful of fresh coriander (cilantro) leaves, finely chopped
a small handful of fresh parsley leaves, finely chopped

I am always keen to experiment with storecupboard spices to create new and exciting flavours and bring more taste and goodness to my dishes. This marinade is probably one of the most versatile and delicious you can make. The ingredients can vary, but normally, roasted cumin and coriander seeds are mixed with saffron, ginger, garlic, paprika and fresh parsley and coriander. Chermoula is a powerful combination of taste and spice equilibrium that originates from North Africa, and the mix definitely evokes the smells and tastes of that region and Moroccan souks and medinas. This can be made in advance and kept in the refrigerator for a few days.

Method

To make the chermoula marinade, heat a small, heavy-based frying pan over a medium heat. Add the cumin and coriander seeds and gently dry-fry for 3–4 minutes until roasted and the aroma is released (be careful that the seeds don't burn). Allow to cool, then grind in a food processor or pestle and mortar into a powder. Place the powder and all the remaining ingredients, including the water from the saffron, in a food processor and blend into a medium-thick paste.

Place the fish on a foil-lined baking tray and spoon over the chermoula paste, spreading it over all sides of each piece of fish. Cover with foil and leave to marinate in the refrigerator for 15–20 minutes.

Preheat a grill to medium.

Remove the foil cover from the fish, place the baking tray under the grill and cook the fish for about 8 minutes. When the fish is cooked, squeeze the juice from the remaining lemon over the fish and serve.

Tips

- Although this recipe is for fish, you can use this marinade for chicken and lamb dishes (if marinating meat, leave the marinade for longer and even overnight to infuse).
- For a delicious vegetarian option, marinate a selection of vegetables and roast with the chermoula paste.

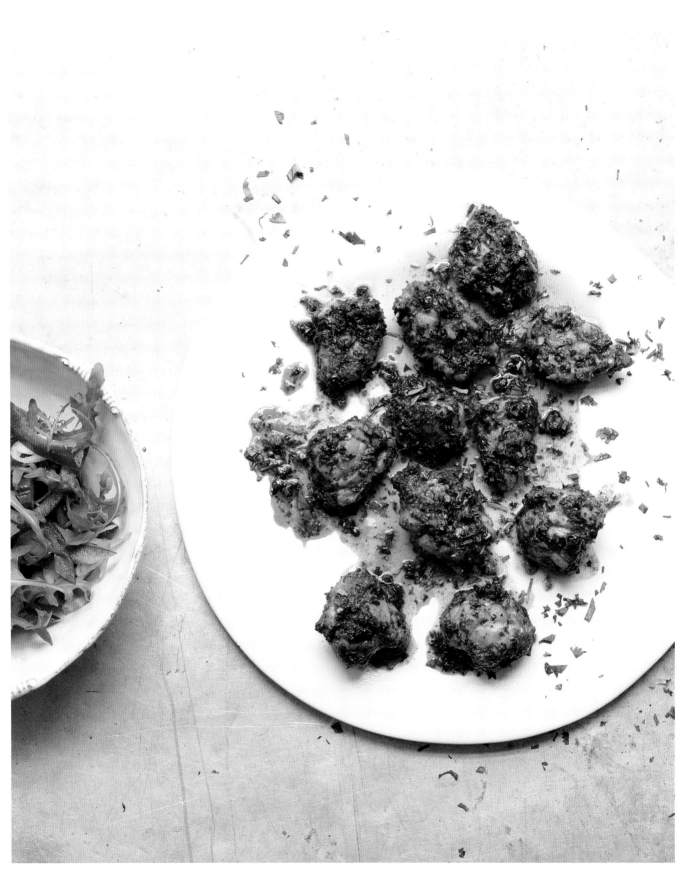

227 KCAL

Sumac-Dusted Hake with Carom Seed Kale

This is a simple to cook dinner dish with a multitude of nutritional benefits. The fish is light, low fat and dusted with sumac. In medieval times, sumac was used to treat many minor ailments, such as stomach complaints, helping to relieve inflammation and for general good health. Sumac adds a wonderful, subtle tangy taste and a crispness to the fish. However, the jewel in the crown in this dish is the carom seeds (they belong to the same family as fennel, anise, dill and caraway). They contain health-promoting essential oils such as thymol, which is known for its antibacterial and anti-fungal properties. We grew up reaching for these seeds whenever we had a stomach bug, felt under the weather or generally queasy. They taste sharp on their own, but in this dish they inject taste into kale, a well-known superfood that is sometimes hard to eat in the quantities we actually need.

Serves 4

Ingredients

For the fish

2 tbsp ground sumac (check it doesn't have any salt added)
1 tsp salt
1 tbsp olive oil
juice of 1 lemon
4 pieces (about 175g/6oz per person) skinned, boned hake or any firm white fish

For the kale

2 tbsp olive oil
1 tbsp carom seeds
5cm/2in piece fresh ginger, peeled and thinly sliced or finely chopped
1 large red onion, peeled and thinly sliced
½ tsp salt
½ small red chilli (medium heat) or ½ tsp chilli (red pepper) flakes (optional)
10–12 cherry tomatoes, cut into quarters
300g/10½oz kale
100g/3½oz spinach leaves

Method

In a small bowl, mix together the sumac, salt, olive oil and half of the lemon juice. Brush onto the fish on both sides and set aside.

For the kale, heat the olive oil in a large wok over a high heat. When the oil is hot, throw in the carom seeds and cook for 1 minute (be careful not to let them burn or they will taste bitter). Add the ginger, red onions and salt and cook over a high heat until the red onion is starting to turn brown, about 2–3 minutes. Do not let them burn or caramelise.

Reduce the heat to medium and carefully add the chilli or flakes (if using) and the tomatoes and cook for 2–3 minutes until the tomatoes are soft. Add the kale, turn up the heat to high and stir-fry for 3–4 minutes, adding 1 tablespoon of water if it's catching on the base of the wok. Stir in the spinach leaves and continue to stir-fry for a further 2–3 minutes until the spinach has wilted. Partially cover and simmer while cooking the fish (you may need to add another sprinkling of hot water if it is sticking).

Preheat the grill to medium.

Place the fish on a non-stick baking tray and grill for 3–4 minutes on each side, crisping one side.

Arrange the kale on a plate and top with the fish. Squeeze the remaining lemon juice over the fish and serve.

Super-Quick Chargrilled Tandoori Tilapia

192 KCAL

Using just a dusting of my Tandoori Spice Rub, you will get a fantastic mix of health-enhancing spices and a massive flavour hit. This mix includes anti-inflammatory and antiseptic turmeric, metabolism-boosting chilli and antioxidant-rich coriander. This is a good lunch or light supper. Eat with my Magnificent Mango Salsa (p.81) for lunch or Cumin and Sumac Sweet Potato Rounds (p.139) for supper.

Method

Preheat the grill to high or heat a barbecue.

Rub the Tandoori Spice Mix over both sides of the fish, then brush the oil over and sprinkle with the salt. Shake the excess rub off the fish and place on a foil-lined grill pan.

Cook the tilapia for 3–4 minutes on each side. When cooked, drizzle with the lime juice and lime zest and serve.

Tip

If you can't find tilapia, then use any light white fish or salmon.

Serves 4

Ingredients

4 tilapia fillets, pin-boned
2 tbsp Tandoori Spice Rub (p.18)
2 tbsp olive oil
½ tsp salt
zest and juice of ½ lime

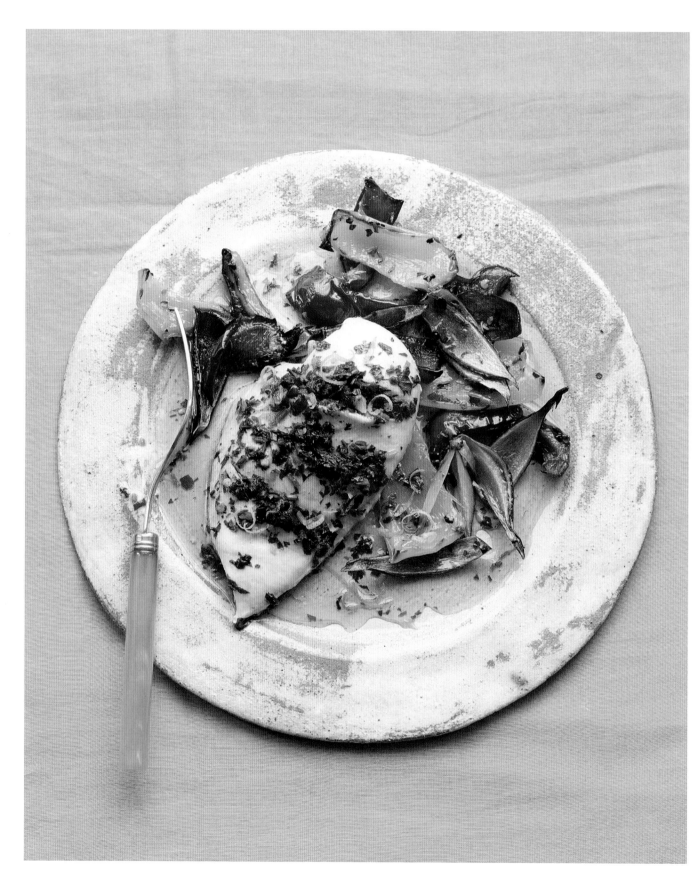

Uplifting Lemon Coriander Chicken with Roasted Peppers

332 KCAL

I love making this dish. It captures the colours of balmy days in the Mediterranean for me. I've taken the traditional Italian gremolata and 'upscaled' it with spices. My version is as fresh but with the addition of tender coriander, ground cumin and chilli flakes so you get a lovely combination of herbs and also healthy spices. The spices lift the taste of the dish and combine together to support the digestion.

Method

Preheat the oven to 220°C/425°F/Gas mark 7.

Start by making the gremolata so that the flavours have time to meld together. Using a pestle and mortar, grind all the ingredients, except the lemon rind, into a rough paste. You can use a food processor but don't blend it too finely. Mix in the lemon rind. Cover and set aside.

Score each chicken breast 2–3 times to make small pockets (do not score all the way through the chicken). Rub salt, pepper and olive oil over the fillets then fill the pockets with equal amounts of the gremolata. Place on an oven tray, cover with foil and cook in the hot oven for 15 minutes. Remove the foil and continue cooking while you prepare the peppers.

Combine all the ingredients for the peppers, except the cumin seeds and oil, in a bowl. Season with a few grinds of black pepper. Place an oven dish or baking tray on the hob, add the olive oil and heat over a medium heat. When the oil is hot, throw in the cumin seeds and cook for 1–2 minutes until the seeds begin to sizzle and release their aroma. Quickly add the ingredients from the bowl. Mix and spread thinly in the oven dish, then place in hot oven on the top rung for 10 minutes. The peppers are ready when they are slightly charred and soft. The chicken and peppers should be ready at the same time. Divide the roasted peppers between plates and top with a piece of chicken.

Tips

- Substitute white fish such as sea bass instead of chicken.
- For a vegetarian option, top a baked sweet potato with the gremolata. I also love the Mediterranean roasted red peppers as a side dish to a lentil bake or just with steamed green vegetables and couscous.
- When cooking the peppers, you need an oven dish or a baking tray that will go on the hob and in the oven.

Serves 4

Ingredients

For the gremolata

zest and juice of 1 large lemon
2 garlic cloves, peeled and roughly chopped
30g/1oz roughly chopped fresh parsley, leaves only
30g/1oz roughly chopped fresh coriander (cilantro)
2 tbsp olive oil
1 tsp roasted ground cumin
1 tsp ground coriander
½ tsp chilli (red pepper) flakes
½ tsp salt

For the chicken

4 skinless, boneless chicken breast fillets
salt and freshly ground black pepper
½ tsp olive oil

For the peppers

2 tbsp olive oil
1 tbsp cumin seeds
2 garlic cloves, peeled and roughly chopped
2 large red onions, peeled and medium sliced
1¼ tsp chilli (red pepper) flakes
¼ tsp salt
freshly ground black pepper
1 red (bell) pepper, deseeded and sliced
1 yellow (bell) pepper, deseeded and sliced

Szechuan Twice-Peppered Prawns

Serves 4

Ingredients

1 tsp Szechuan peppercorns
¾ tsp salt crystals
1 tsp black peppercorns
255g/9oz raw peeled king prawns (shrimp)
2 tbsp groundnut (peanut) oil
a large squeeze of lemon

I was really astonished when I first tried Szechuan peppercorns, as the instant tingling and lively citrus taste is really unusual. Szechuan pepper has been around for centuries in Asia. My first experience of this dish was in a noisy Hong Kong night street food market. What a place!! I don't think there's a place like it on earth and as an 18-year-old, I couldn't believe that everything I wanted to eat was there alive in front of me and I could pick it and have it cooked right there and then (including these enormous prawns). This is a simple and speedy dish with Szechuan pepper and deep, dark flavoured black peppercorns. Szechuan pepper actually comes from a berry and black peppercorns come from India and the Indian sub-continent but they are both good for calming the digestion.

This light and easy supper dish is good to eat with my Simple Vermicelli Salad (see p.126).

Method

Place the Szechuan peppers, salt and black peppercorns in a pestle and mortar or electric grinder and grind into a fine powder. If using a pestle and mortar, sieve the mixture to remove any husks.

Pat the prawns dry and mix in the pepper and salt mixture.

Heat a non-stick frying pan over a medium-high heat and add the oil. When the oil is hot, add the prawns and cook for 2–3 minutes on each side until they turn pink. When cooked, squeeze a little fresh lemon over the top and serve.

Tips

• Squid is also good for this recipe.
• For a vegetarian version, use firm tofu, cut into cubes.

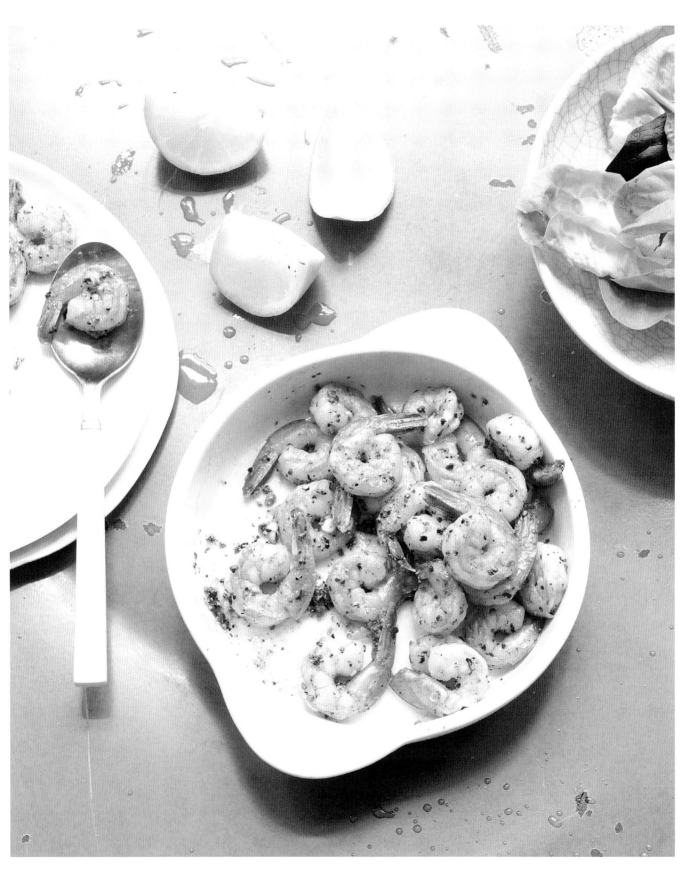

Thai-Spiced Seared Tuna with Fennel and Blood Orange Salad

Serves 4

Ingredients

a small bunch of fresh basil leaves,
　save a few leaves to garnish
4 blood oranges

1 medium mild red chilli,
　finely chopped
5 tbsp olive oil
salt and freshly ground
　black pepper
2 fennel bulbs
5cm/2in piece fresh ginger,
　peeled and grated
2 tsp rice wine vinegar or mirin
1 tsp chilli (red pepper) flakes
2 tbsp soy sauce
4 medium tuna steaks, about
　175g/6oz each
2 tsp fennel seeds, lightly toasted

This is a simple and refreshing salad balancing citrus flavour with the meaty, spicy taste of the seared tuna – beautiful, aromatic and zingy. The ginger adds a gentle heat and is balanced for your digestion by the warm fennel seeds at the end.

Method

For the dressing, roughly chop the basil leaves, place in a bowl and add the juice and zest of 1 of the blood oranges. Add the red chilli, 3 tablespoons olive oil and salt and pepper to taste. Mix together well and set aside.

Peel the remaining blood oranges, carefully slicing them so you achieve wheel-like slices. Thinly slice the fennel and arrange on a plate with the blood orange slices. Mix the dressing and pour over the orange and fennel, then allow to infuse while preparing the tuna.

In a separate bowl (large enough for the tuna steaks to marinate in), mix the ginger, rice wine, chilli flakes, soy sauce and remaining olive oil together. Dip the tuna steaks in and turn until they are coated with the marinade. Cover and leave for 5–10 minutes, but no longer or the fish will begin to break down.

Heat a non-stick pan until hot. One or two at a time, sear the tuna steaks in the hot pan – only 1–2 minutes on each side – taking care not to overcook the fish. They should be seared on the outside but not cooked all the way through. Slice each steak into 2.5cm/1in slices and arrange over the fennel and orange salad. Sprinkle over the toasted fennel seeds and the remaining basil leaves before serving immediately.

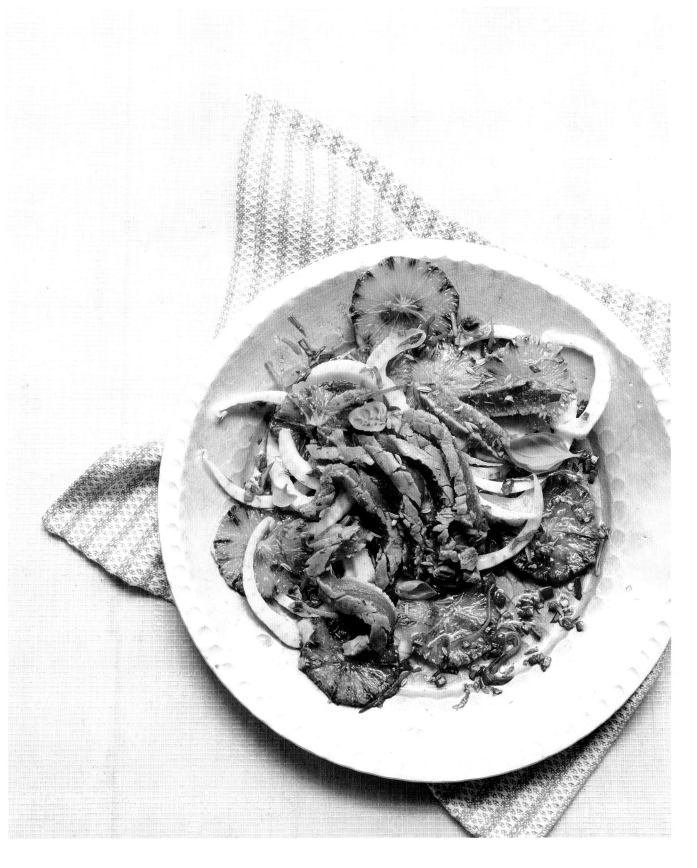

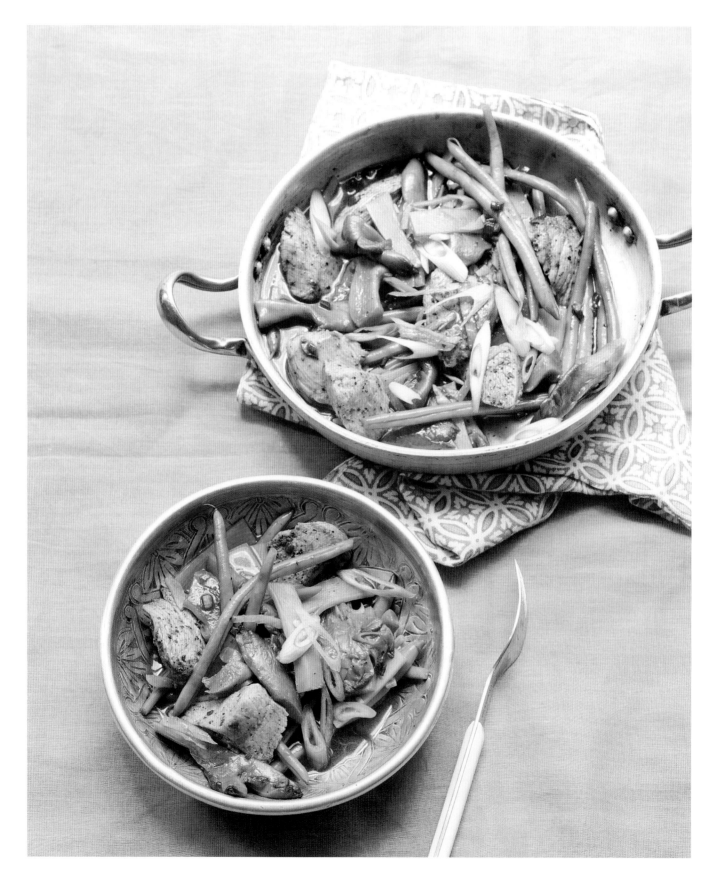

Szechuan-Style Chicken and Green Beans

256 KCAL

I love having a Chinese takeaway, but more often than not, they are oily and full of fat. Of course, these takeaway dishes aren't always executed faithfully to the original dish, so I have peeled back this dish using traditional spices and ingredients. My Szechuan Spice Rub includes authentic Chinese spices (Szechuan pepper, star anise, fennel seeds, cloves, black peppercorns and cinnamon) which have been used since the beginning of Chinese medicinal history to promote health and to stave off ailments while nourishing our bodies.

Method

Put the chicken pieces in a bowl and sprinkle the Szechuan-Style Spice Rub and rice wine over. Cover and set aside while preparing the vegetables.

Heat a large wok over a very high heat and add the groundnut oil. Throw in the ginger, garlic and chilli, and after 30 seconds (do not brown) add the green beans. Stir-fry over a high heat for 3–4 minutes, then add in the chicken and stir-fry for a further 2–3 minutes. Add the mushrooms and bamboo shoots and stir-fry for 2 minutes. Season with the soy sauce and sesame oil. Pour in the stock and bring quickly to the boil then add the cornflour. The chicken should be cooked but keep the green beans *al dente*. Check the seasoning, you may need to add ½ teaspoon salt depending on how salty the soy sauce is. Sprinkle the spring onions over the top and serve.

Tips

- Marinating the chicken before cooking tenderises it.
- For a vegetarian option, use firm tofu grilled in cubes and added to the dish instead of the chicken, then remove it after 2–3 minutes and add it back in at the end of cooking.

Serves 4

Ingredients

- 4 medium skinless, boneless chicken breasts, sliced into 2.5cm/1in strips
- 1 tbsp Szechuan-Style Spice Rub (see p.19)
- ½ tsp rice wine or mirin
- 2 tbsp groundnut (peanut) oil
- 2.5cm/1in piece fresh ginger, peeled and sliced or grated
- 2 garlic cloves, peeled and crushed
- 1 medium chilli, finely chopped
- 200g/7oz green beans, trimmed and kept whole
- 100g/3½oz oyster mushrooms, thickly sliced
- 60g/2¼oz bamboo shoots
- 2 tbsp light soy sauce
- ½ tsp sesame oil
- 400ml/14fl oz/1¾ cups hot low-salt chicken or vegetable stock (broth)
- 1 tbsp cornflour (cornstarch) mixed with 2 tbsp cold water
- 4 spring onions (scallions), cut thinly on the bias

Punjabi Jeera Chicken (Cumin Chicken)

Serves 4

Ingredients

2 garlic cloves, peeled and cut in half

5cm/2in piece fresh ginger, peeled and roughly chopped

15g/½oz fresh coriander (cilantro) including stems (leave a few leaves for the garnish)

3 green chillies (for medium heat)

½ tsp salt

3 tbsp olive oil

600g/1lb 5oz chicken thighs, skinned and boned or chicken breast, any fat removed and cut into 5cm/2in pieces

1 tbsp cumin seeds

1 large red onion, peeled and sliced

1 tbsp roasted ground cumin

a squeeze of lemon (optional)

A classic North Indian family dish, this is one of my family's signature dishes and we eat it at all our celebratory events. The delicious taste belies the simplicity of it. Whole cumin seeds and ground roasted cumin are the main spices, with the addition of a little chilli for an extra bite. Cumin is a legendary spice dating back centuries and is rich in antioxidants, iron, and calms and soothes the digestive system.

Method

In a food processor, combine the garlic, ginger, coriander and green chillies and blitz until finely chopped. Mix in the salt and 1 tablespoon olive oil to make a paste and pour into a bowl. Add the chicken pieces to the paste and mix thoroughly so the chicken is coated all over. Cover and chill in the refrigerator for 10–15 minutes, or up to 1 hour.

Preheat the oven to 200°C/400°F/Gas mark 6.

Heat a large ovenproof baking tray on the hob over a medium heat and add the remaining olive oil. When the oil is hot, throw in the cumin seeds and, as soon as they start to sizzle, add the sliced onion and the chicken with all of the paste. Turn, coating the chicken well for 3–4 minutes, or until the chicken begins to brown, then cook in the hot oven for 5–7 minutes. Take the tray out and sprinkle with the ground cumin and return to the oven for a further 5–6 minutes, or until the chicken is cooked.

Garnish with a few coriander leaves and a squeeze of lemon to serve.

Tips

- I usually use skinned chicken wings, but as these are hard to find except in some Asian butchers, I have substituted boneless and skinless chicken thighs. You can use chicken breast instead.
- To roast cumin seeds, I roast them in a dry frying pan over a medium heat for 4–5 minutes until lightly brown. Keep moving them so they don't burn. Transfer them to a pestle and mortar and grind to a fine powder.
- I eat this dish with salad, such as my Mooli Slaw (p.94) and Cucumber and Mint Raita (p.143). This also goes well with my Shaved Fennel, Fennel Seeds, Cucumber and Pomegranate Side (p.138).

Rose Petal Ras el Hanout Red Snapper

163 KCAL

When I open my spice box and smell the aroma of ras el hanout, I'm transported back to the bustling markets in Morocco full of alluring, colourful mounds of spices. Ras el hanout encapsulates sweetness, savouriness and spiciness in one spice mix! It is a veritable Pandora's box of spices – sometimes over 20 spices go into this mix. The good news is that they are all warming, nutritious spices and include cumin, coriander, cinnamon and ginger. For this recipe, look for the variety with rose petals as this adds a depth and gives this dish a lovely intensity.

Serves 4

Ingredients

3 tbsp plain yogurt
zest and juice of ½ lemon
1 tsp ras el hanout
4 red snapper fillets
a large handful of fresh coriander (cilantro), roughly chopped
1 large onion, peeled and sliced
salt, to taste (check your ras el hanout isn't already salted)

Method

In a bowl, mix the yogurt with the lemon, lemon zest and ras el hanout. Place the fish in this mixture and turn the fish gently until it is coated. Cover and leave in the refrigerator for 10 minutes but not longer than 1 hour. Sprinkle with the chopped coriander.

Preheat the oven to 180°C/350°F/Gas mark 4.

Place the sliced onion on a large piece of foil paper (large enough to fold over the top). Place the fish on the onion slices, then bring the 2 sides of the foil together to form a parcel and close lightly. Place the parcel on an oven tray and bake in the hot oven for 8–10 minutes until cooked.

Open the parcel carefully and serve with the liquid which has formed in the foil paper.

Tip

I eat this with my Fennel, Cucumber and Pomegranate Salad (p.138).

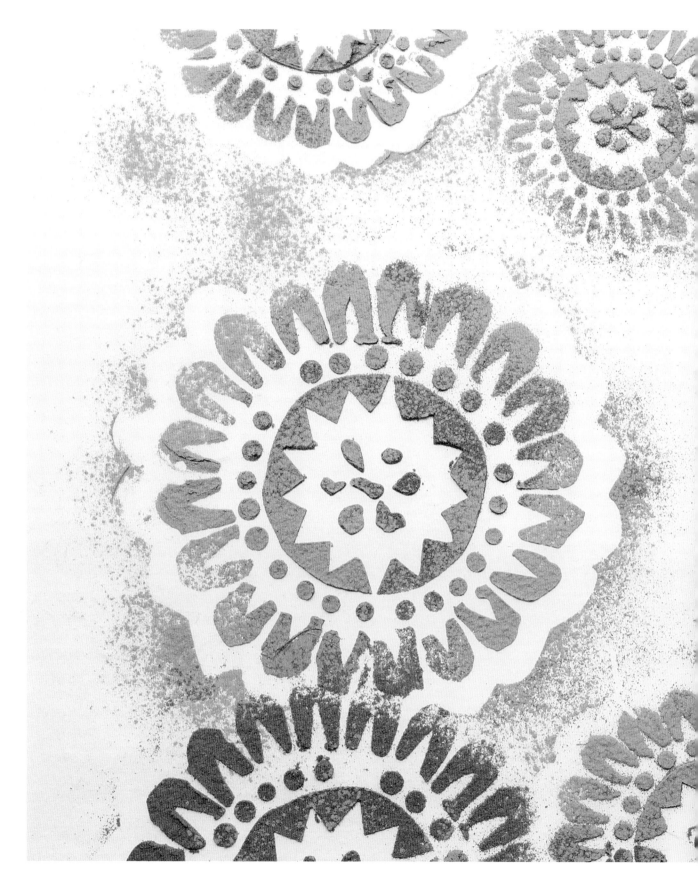

Meals to Share and to Impress

For me, sharing a meal with friends and family is not only a very social thing to do, it is also a healthy way of eating as I believe that enjoying food while you eat it sends positive signals to the digestion and helps to absorb all the good vitamins and nutrients from the food. Also, sharing an exciting meal, which you have cooked and spent time over, is a lovely way of demonstrating how much you love and care for your friends and family.

The meals in this chapter are easy to cook but look and taste impressive. You can excite your friends with a selection of contemporary dishes from around the world. There is a mix of Asian, Middle Eastern and Mediterranean-inspired dishes.

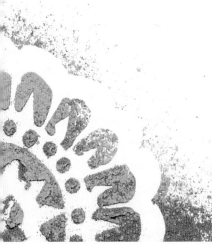

An Indian Abroad Sunday Roast

Serves 4

Ingredients

1 medium free-range chicken,
  about 1.5kg/3lb 5oz, skinned
2 large onions, peeled,
  cut 1 in half and 1 into quarters
1 whole head of garlic, cut in half
100ml/3½fl oz/½ cup hot water

For the marinade

2 garlic cloves, peeled
5cm/2in piece fresh ginger,
  peeled
1 green chilli, roughly chopped
a small bunch of fresh coriander
  (cilantro), roughly chopped
1 large lemon
1 tsp salt
3 tbsp olive oil
150g/5¼oz/⅔ cup plain yogurt
2½ tbsp Tandoori Spice Rub (p.18)
½ tsp chilli powder (optional)

Tip

Marinate the chicken for as long as possible – 4–6 hours in the refrigerator is good or even overnight. Ask your butcher to skin the chicken if you don't want to do this yourself.

As a family we love to make a 'traditional' English roast but we can't help introducing extra flavour through spices to each of the dishes. Using your Tandoori Spice Rub, you can bring together the traditional Sunday roast with the essence of India, enjoy a change in taste and also gain extra health benefits from the spices (and 'superfoods' garlic and ginger). When we make Indian chicken, we almost always remove the skin – this is easy to do if you follow the instructions in the recipe and it will also allow the marinade to really infuse the chicken.

As the chicken is so succulent and filling, it doesn't need many 'sides' and I often eat this with a cucumber raita or if it's for a big family gathering, with Cumin and Sumac Sweet Potato Rounds (p.139).

Method

To make the marinade, put the garlic, ginger, green chilli, coriander, juice of ½ the lemon, salt and olive oil in a food processor and pulse to a paste. This can also be done in a large pestle and mortar. Place the paste in a bowl and mix in the yogurt, Spice Rub and chilli powder (if using).

Using a very sharp knife, cut down the middle of the breastbone of the chicken. Separate the skin and pull off. To skin the drumsticks, cut around the bottom of the leg then cut the skin up the leg and gently pull off. Turn the chicken over and do the same. There's no need to skin the wings.

Make deep slashes into the breast and legs of the chicken, then rub the marinade deep into the slashes. Place an onion half and the remaining lemon half in the cavity of the chicken. Cover loosely with foil and place in the refrigerator to marinate (see tip below).

Preheat the oven to 180°C/350°F/Gas mark 4.

Remove the chicken from the refrigerator and place the 4 onion halves and whole garlic head pieces on the base of a large oven tray. Seat the chicken on the top. Pour the hot water in the bottom of the tray. Cover the chicken loosely with foil and cook in the hot oven, regularly basting with the juice. Ten minutes before the chicken is ready, remove the foil and continue cooking until the juices run clear when a skewer is inserted into the thickest part of the meat. When cooked, take the chicken out of the oven, loosely wrap with foil and allow to rest for 10–15 minutes before serving.

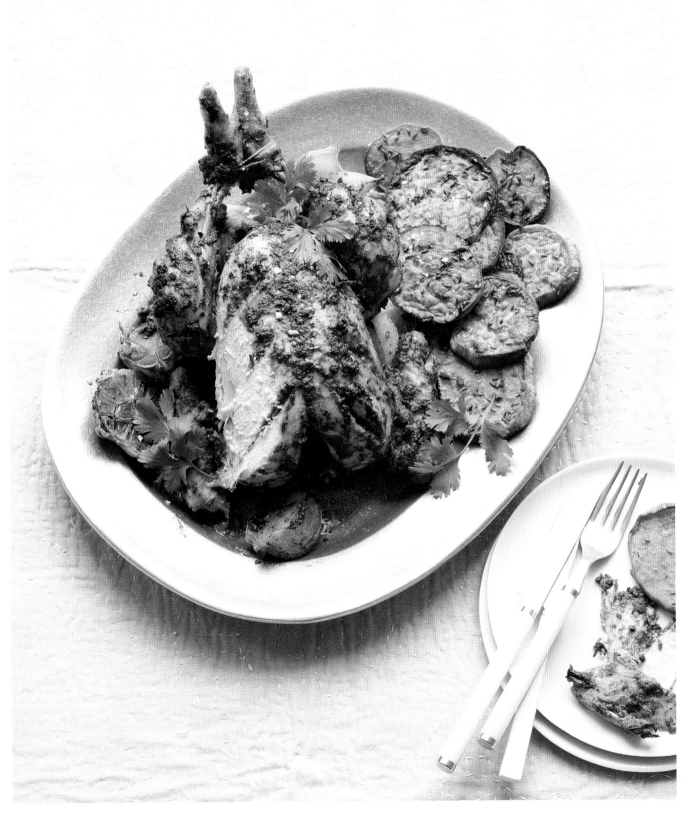

Magic Beans and Skinny Paneer

Serves 4

Ingredients

2 tbsp olive oil

1 tsp grated fresh ginger

1–2 green chillies, finely chopped (1 for a mild taste and 2 for medium hot)

1 tsp ground turmeric

1 tsp ground coriander

½ tsp salt

200g/7oz can chopped tomatoes

225g/8oz purple French (green), runner (string) or flat beans, cut into 1cm/½in pieces

2 tbsp warm water

a small handful of fresh coriander (cilantro) leaves, roughly chopped

For the paneer

1.5 litres/2½ pints/6⅓ cups semi-skimmed (low-fat) cow's milk

¼ tsp salt

3 tbsp lemon juice

These purple French beans are a feast for the eyes and turn green when cooked, so are fun ingredients to use. Here, they are combined with a low-fat version of paneer, which is itself a rather magical Indian food. By just combining separated milk and lemon, you can quickly create a wonderful creamy cheese, which is a real treat. Paneer is high in protein and great at absorbing flavours, so I have added ginger, chilli, turmeric and ground coriander for flavour and nutrition.

Method

Bring the milk to the boil in a large saucepan over a gentle heat. Add the salt and stir constantly. As it starts to boil, quickly take it off the heat and pour in the lemon juice. Stir and you will see that the milk solids and the whey will begin to separate. Set aside for 5–10 minutes.

Line a colander with muslin cloth, leaving enough cloth hanging over the sides so that you can gather them together. Carefully pour in the milk and bring the cloth together to cover. Leave to stand for 10–15 minutes then squeeze out the excess water. The paneer should have the consistency of cottage cheese.

Heat a large wok or a sauté pan over a medium heat and add the olive oil. When the oil is hot, add the ginger and green chilli and let it sizzle for 2 minutes. Add the turmeric, coriander and salt, and cook for 1–2 minutes. Add the tomatoes and the juice from the can and cook over a medium heat for 4–5 minutes. Add the purple beans and continue cooking until the beans are soft. If the mixture is sticking, then add the warm water.

When the beans are soft, carefully crumble in the paneer and coat with the mixture. Cover with a lid and simmer for 5 minutes. Sprinkle the chopped coriander over the paneer before serving.

Tips

- Freshly made paneer is soft and crumbly and has the consistency of cottage cheese. After a couple of hours, it will harden and it can then be cut into cubes. I like to make double the quantity as it keeps in an airtight container in the refrigerator for 3–4 days and then I can make this dish again or eat it with a salad instead of feta.
- You will need a muslin cloth or a very sheer tea towel.

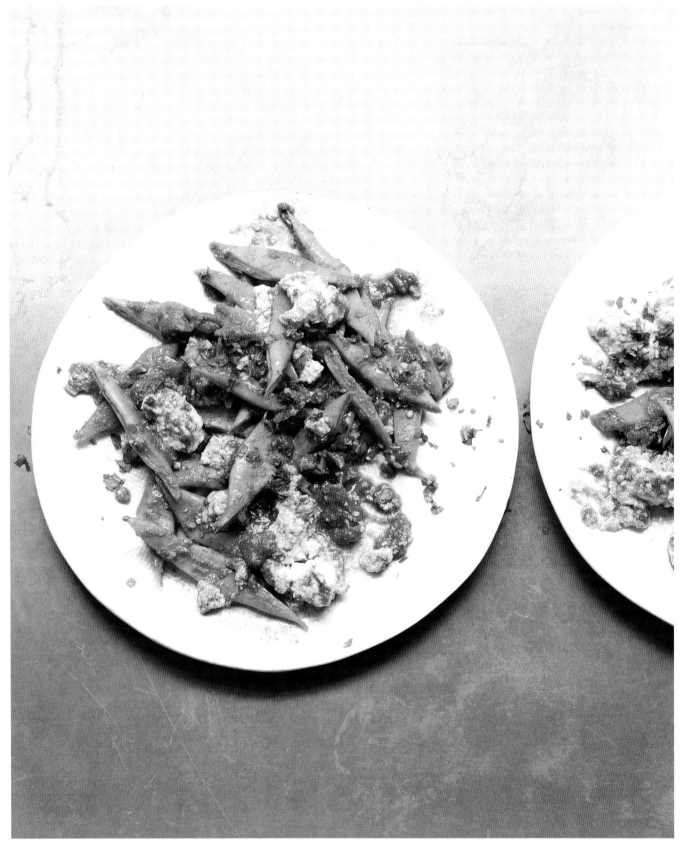

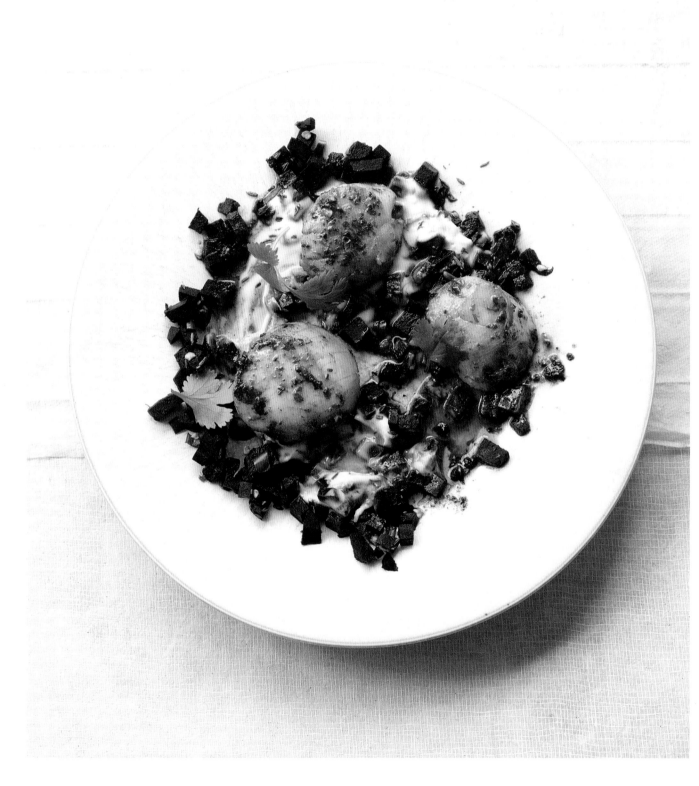

Lime, Chilli and Coriander Scallops on a Bed of Cumin-Spiced Beetroot

204 KCAL

This is not only a beautiful dish, but the soft, hot and spicy scallops are complemented perfectly by the cool, creamy beetroot. The roasted cumin adds aroma, depth and a feeling of restorative energy. The marinade can be made and kept for a couple of days in the refrigerator in a sealed container (it does improve too). If you don't have time to roast the cumin seeds, buy good ground cumin instead.

Method

Warm a small pan over a medium heat. Throw in the cumin seeds and gently dry-fry for 2–3 minutes until the seeds are slightly brown (you will smell it roasting). Place the seeds in a pestle and mortar and grind to a powder, or use an electric grinder.

Grate the beetroot into a bowl and add the garlic and a quarter of the chopped chilli. Add the yogurt and a third of the ground cumin to the beetroot and mix well. Leave to stand for 10–15 minutes while preparing the scallops.

In a large pestle and mortar or an electric chopper, place the remaining chilli, the coriander, including the stems as they add extra flavour, 1 tablespoon olive oil, juice of ½ lime, the remaining ground cumin, the turmeric, chilli powder and water, and chop until a thick paste is formed. Place the paste in a bowl, stir in the lime zest and fold in the scallops. Cover and leave to marinate in the refrigerator for 5–10 minutes – no longer.

Spoon a quarter of the beetroot mixture on to each plate.

Heat the remaining olive oil in a non-stick pan over a medium heat. When the oil is hot, add the scallops in small batches (do not crowd the pan as you want to colour the scallops and not lose the marinade paste) and cook quickly, about 1–2 minutes on each side (they turn opaque when cooked – take care not to overcook). Transfer them to a warm plate and, when all of them are cooked, arrange them over each dollop of beetroot mixture on the plates. Squeeze a little of the remaining lime over each scallop and sprinkle some roughly chopped coriander leaves across the dish.

Serves 4

Ingredients

3 tbsp cumin seeds
250g/9oz (about 2 large) cooked beetroot, peeled
1 small garlic clove, peeled and crushed
1 large red chilli, roughly chopped
150g/5¼oz/⅔ cup plain live yogurt
12 scallops, lightly washed and patted dry
a large bunch of fresh coriander (cilantro), including the stems, leave a small amount to sprinkle over the scallops when serving
3 tbsp olive oil
zest and juice of 1 lime
½ tsp ground turmeric
½ tsp chilli powder
4 tbsp water

Tip

This marinade is also delicious with chicken pieces (add 2 finely chopped garlic cloves if using chicken) instead of the scallops.

315 KCAL

Chinese Pork Tenderloin with Braised Pak Choi and Baby Leeks

Serves 4

Ingredients

450g/1lb pork tenderloin, sliced into 8 medallions, each 2.5cm/1in thick

For the marinade

2 garlic cloves, peeled and finely chopped
2 tbsp Szechuan-Style Spice Rub (see p.19)
1 tbsp dark soy sauce
1 tbsp honey
1 tbsp lemon juice
1 tsp sesame oil
1 tsp chilli (red pepper) flakes
2 tbsp olive oil

For the braised pak choi with baby leeks

2 tbsp vegetable oil
5cm/2in piece fresh ginger, peeled and shredded
135g/5oz baby leeks, trimmed and sliced in half
125g/4½oz spring onions (scallions), roughly chopped
300g/10½oz pak choi, leaves separated and trimmed
1 small red chilli, finely chopped (optional)
2 tbsp soy sauce
2 tbsp warm water
a pinch of salt
½ tsp ground white pepper

Pork tenderloin has no fat and is very lean, but this means that it does need help to give it flavour. Using your Szechuan-Style Spice Rub (flavoured with star anise, fennel, cloves, Szechuan peppercorns and cinnamon) to marinate this cut will give the meat taste. The ingredients in this rub are a cornucopia of goodness as each spice is nutritious in its own right and when mixed together pack a big punch. Pak choi with baby leeks is a lovely vegetable side and combined with warming ginger acts as a healthy support dish to the pork, too.

Method

In a bowl, mix together all the ingredients for the marinade. Brush the marinade over each medallion on both sides, then cover and leave in the refrigerator for 15–30 minutes.

Preheat the oven to 180°C/350°F/Gas mark 4.

For the braised pak choi and baby leeks, heat the oil in a wok over a medium heat. When the oil is hot, add the ginger and mix for 1 minute then quickly add the baby leeks, spring onions, pak choi and chilli (if using). Pour in the soy sauce and water and stir-fry for 2 minutes. Reduce the heat to low, cover and cook for 4–5 minutes, or until the vegetables are cooked. Season with the salt and pepper and mix to combine.

Place the medallions on a baking tray and cook for 4–5 minutes on each side until cooked. Do not overcook. Serve with the braised pak choi and baby leeks.

Tip

You can also use this marinade for chicken.

Moroccan Cinnamon and Preserved Lemon Chicken

322 KCAL

Charting my eating life, one of my most exciting moments came when I was introduced to Middle Eastern herbs and spices. Of course, these spices have been used in dishes in the Middle East for centuries and the striking taste was what first attracted me, but as I delved deeper, I found that these spices were also used for their extensive health properties. Cinnamon, saffron and ginger all have strong flavours as well as calmative and health-giving properties. Turmeric is a super-spice as it contains a compound called curcumin, which has powerful anti-inflammatory effects and is a very strong antioxidant. So, fantastic taste and healthy! This dish can be made in a traditional tagine or a large, heavy-based casserole or even slow cooked in the oven.

Method

Cut off any fat (chicken thighs can be fatty, but work better for this dish than chicken breast which can taste dry after this length of time cooking).

In a large bowl, combine all the ingredients for the marinade (including the water and the stems from the saffron) and mix in the chicken. Mix well so that the chicken is covered in the marinade. Cover and leave to marinate in the refrigerator for at least 2 hours, or overnight.

Heat the olive oil in a large pan over a medium heat. When the oil is hot, add the chicken, only not the marinade (set the marinade aside), and cook for 2–3 minutes. Add the onions and the 1 tablespoon Moroccan Spice Rub and stir for 1–2 minutes. Add the marinade and lemon peel and cook for 1 minute, then add the herbs and chicken stock. Bring to the boil then reduce the heat to a simmer. Sprinkle over the paprika and cook for 30–40 minutes in a tagine or a medium-hot oven. You should have a thick sauce; if it is starting to look dry, add 1–2 tablespoons hot water. After this time, add the olives and cook for a further 5 minutes. Mix in the remaining parsley and coriander leaves, check the seasoning, and serve with warm couscous to soak up all the juices.

Tips

- For a vegetarian option, you can substitute the chicken with precooked chickpeas (400g/14oz) and ½ large butternut squash, cut into cubes.
- If you are gluten intolerant you can buy gluten-free couscous made from millet, or use quinoa, which goes very well with this recipe.

Serves 4

Ingredients

4 medium or 6 small chicken thighs, skinned and on the bone is better for this dish, washed well and patted dry

3 tbsp olive oil

1 large onion, peeled and roughly sliced

1 tbsp Moroccan Spice Rub (p.19)

2 preserved lemons, pulp from the lemons scooped out and discarded and peel finely chopped

a small bunch of fresh parsley, roughly chopped, plus 1 tbsp to garnish

a small bunch of fresh coriander (cilantro), roughly chopped, plus 1 tbsp to garnish

720ml/1¼ pints/3¼ cups hot low-salt chicken stock (broth)

½ tsp paprika powder

56g/2oz/⅓ cup green olives (no oil)

For the marinade

3 garlic cloves, peeled and finely chopped

6–7 saffron threads, crushed and soaked in 4 tbsp hot water for 5 minutes

2 tbsp Moroccan Spice Rub (see p.19)

1 tsp chilli (red pepper) flakes

juice of ½ lemon

½ tsp salt

Prawn Cocktail – Hanoi Style with Vermicelli Salad

Serves 4

Ingredients

For the prawns

1 tbsp coriander seeds or 1 tsp ground coriander
400g/14oz raw tiger prawns (shrimp), peeled, deveined and heads removed
1 tsp ground turmeric
½ tsp salt
2 garlic cloves, finely chopped
½ medium red chilli, finely sliced
3 tbsp lime juice
2 tbsp olive oil
⅓ cos lettuce, finely shredded
1 large carrot, grated
½ red onion, finely sliced

For the tamarind sauce

2 tbsp tamarind paste
4 tsp warm water
½ tsp palm sugar
½ tsp ground ginger
½ tsp ground cumin

For the vermicelli salad

200g/7oz rice noodles
15g/½oz fresh coriander (cilantro) leaves, roughly chopped
15g/½oz fresh Thai basil leaves, roughly chopped
5g/⅛oz fresh mint leaves, roughly chopped
2 spring onions (scallions), roughly chopped
a sprinkling of toasted peanuts

Hanoi is a wonderful city of contrasts – from families cooking their meals on the pavements on small burners to swanky restaurants serving sophisticated dishes. We went to a lovely restaurant (we loved it so much, we went twice!) and had this starter. I loved the taste of the lightly spiced prawns in a sour tamarind sauce and it was playfully served in long shot glasses. I have added to this dish so it can be eaten as a special lunch or a filling dinner. The prawns are stir-fried simply in turmeric, crushed roasted coriander seeds and a touch of red chilli, then placed in a glass with shredded lettuce, julienned carrots and onion on a tangy tamarind sauce. Turmeric will boost your immune system and coriander seeds will not only add a distinctive and light citrus flavour, but they are also a good source of minerals and vitamin C. Served with a delicious and healthy vermicelli salad, it is a fun dish – fun to make, share and eat.

Method

Heat a small frying pan over a medium heat. When hot, add the coriander seeds and roast for 3–4 minutes until the aroma is released. Place the seeds in an electric grinder or pestle and mortar and grind into a powder (not too fine).

Place the prawns in a large bowl and sprinkle over the turmeric, coriander, salt, garlic, chilli and lime juice. Mix together, cover and set aside for 10 minutes.

Mix the tamarind paste and warm water together. Strain to remove any lumps or bits or the tamarind seed, then warm in a small saucepan. Mix in the sugar, ginger and cumin, and warm for 2–3 minutes until the sugar is dissolved. It should form a thick paste.

Prepare high-ball glasses by arranging the lettuce, carrots and onion slices in layers. Add a small dollop of the tamarind sauce to each glass.

Heat the olive oil in a non-stick pan or wok. When the oil is very hot, add the prawns and stir-fry until cooked.

Place equal amounts of the prawns on top of each glass.

To make the vermicelli salad, make the dressing by warming all the ingredients together gently in a saucepan.

Cook the noodles according to the packet instructions, then place on a serving plate and pour over the dressing. Sprinkle the herbs and spring onions over the noodles and mix well. Sprinkle over the roasted peanuts and serve with the prawn cocktail.

Tips

- For a vegetarian option, use cubed tofu instead of the prawns.
- You can use 1 teaspoon ground coriander if you don't have seeds.
- The vermicelli salad also goes well with the Saigon-Style Fillet of Beef (p.129).

For the dressing

100ml/3½fl oz/½ cup warm
   water
2 tbsp soy sauce
½ tsp finely chopped
   fresh ginger
2 tbsp olive oil
½ tsp sesame oil
½ chopped red chilli
½ tsp fish sauce
juice of ½ lime
 a pinch of palm sugar

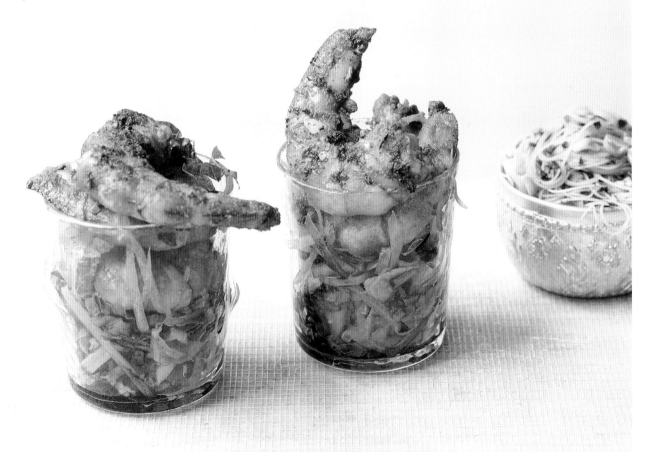

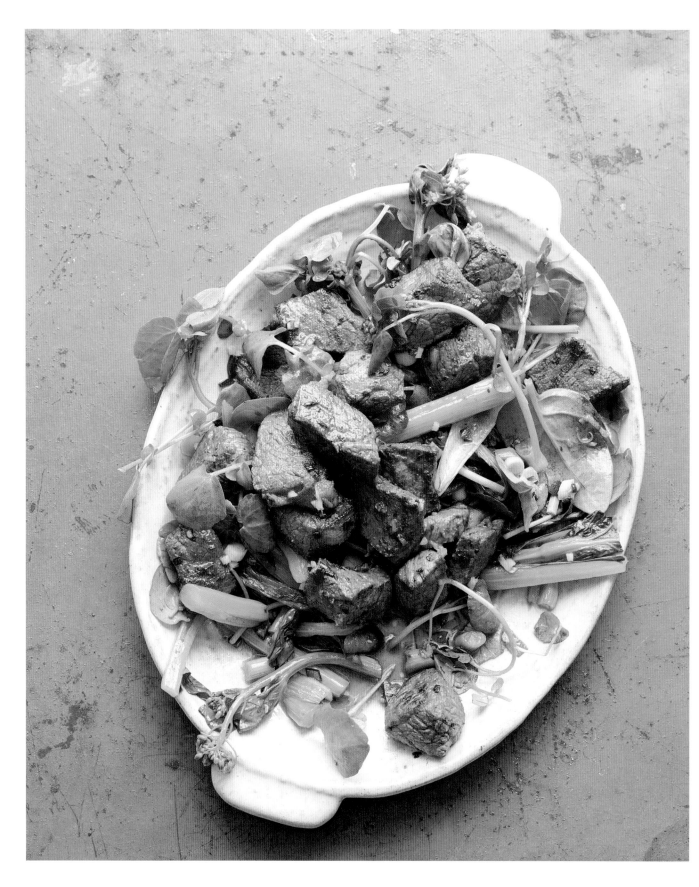

Saigon-Style Fillet of Beef

267 KCAL

I enjoyed this dish so much when I was in Saigon – officially Ho Chi Minh City, but most of the locals still call it Saigon. Succulent, tender cubes of beef, marinated in turmeric and garlic, served with a warm wilted ginger and chilli watercress, pak choi and spring onion salad – light but satisfying and great to share for a special dinner. The salad quantities look big but will wilt down. Beef fillet is extravagant, but it is definitely worth it in this dish.

Method

Combine the olive oil, salt, garlic, turmeric and chilli flakes in a bowl and mix in the beef cubes. Cover and leave to marinate in the refrigerator for 15–20 minutes.

Put the watercress, spinach, choi sam and the spring onions on a large plate.

To make the salad dressing, heat the olive oil in a pan. When the oil is warm, add the ginger, soy sauce, fish sauce, red chilli, orange zest and water and cook over a gentle heat for 2 minutes. Mix in the orange juice, set aside while cooking the beef, then pour the warm dressing over the vegetables and gently toss together.

Heat a non-stick frying pan. When pan is very hot, shake the marinade off the beef and add the beef to the pan. Cook the beef to your taste – medium rare is good. When ready, place the beef and any juices from the pan onto the vegetables and drizzle over the lime juice and black pepper. Serve immediately.

Tips

- For a vegetarian option, try this dish with marinated silken tofu or even portobello mushrooms, sliced and marinated as in the recipe.
- This dish goes very well with my Hanoi-Style Vermicelli Salad (p.126) if you are entertaining.

Serves 4

Ingredients

For the beef

1 tbsp olive oil
¼ tsp salt
2 garlic cloves, peeled and finely chopped
1 tsp ground turmeric
1 tsp chilli (red pepper) flakes
400g/14oz beef fillet, cut into cubes
juice of 1 small lime
a few grinds of black pepper

For the warm salad

200g/7oz watercress
200g/7oz baby spinach leaves
200g/7oz choi sam or pak choi, roughly chopped
4 spring onions (scallions), finely chopped

For the salad dressing

2 tbsp olive oil
5cm/2in piece fresh ginger, peeled and finely chopped
1 tbsp light soy sauce
1 tbsp fish sauce
1 medium red chilli, chopped
zest and juice of 1 orange
2 tbsp warm water

Steaming Mexican Seasoned Mussels

Serves 4

Ingredients

1kg/2¼1b fresh mussels

2 tbsp olive oil

2 garlic cloves, peeled and finely chopped

5 eschalion shallots, peeled and finely chopped

1 red ancho chilli, finely chopped, or use ½ tsp smoked paprika

1½ tbsp Mexican Spice Rub (p.18)

200g/7oz can chopped tomatoes

150g/5¼oz chestnut (cremini) or button (white) mushrooms, thinly sliced

1 litre/1¾ pints/4 cups low-salt chicken or vegetable stock (broth)

salt

juice of 1 lime

a large handful of fresh parsley leaves, roughly chopped

I love experimenting with my spice rubs and combining them with the foods I like to eat. So, here's my lovely sharing and entertaining dish made easy with my Mexican Spice Rub full of good, healthy spices and fantastic flavour. The spices add a nutritional punch to the mussels. When you lift the lid on the mussels, the full aroma of the spice mix will hit you, and I guarantee that you won't be able to eat these fast enough! To make it extra healthy, I am using stock instead of wine.

Method

Prepare the mussels by washing under a cold tap to remove any grit or dirt. Pull out any beards, taking care not to disturb the mussels. Discard any that are open.

Heat the olive oil in a large pan over a medium heat. Add the garlic, shallots and chilli, and cook for 2–3 minutes until soft. Add the Mexican Spice Rub, stir for 1 minute, then add the tomatoes and mushrooms and cook for 4–5 minutes. Pour in the stock and bring to the boil. Reduce the heat to medium, taste the sauce and season with salt, if needed, and simmer for 2–3 minutes.

Stir in the mussels and the lime juice. Cover with a lid and allow the mussels to steam for about 8–10 minutes, or until all the mussels have opened. Shake the pan. Discard any unopened mussels. Sprinkle in the parsley, then ladle into bowls and serve steaming hot.

Tips

- It would be good to eat this with corn bread or corn tortillas, but I like to eat them with sourdough bread too.
- The ancho chilli is optional but it does add a deep smoky flavour.

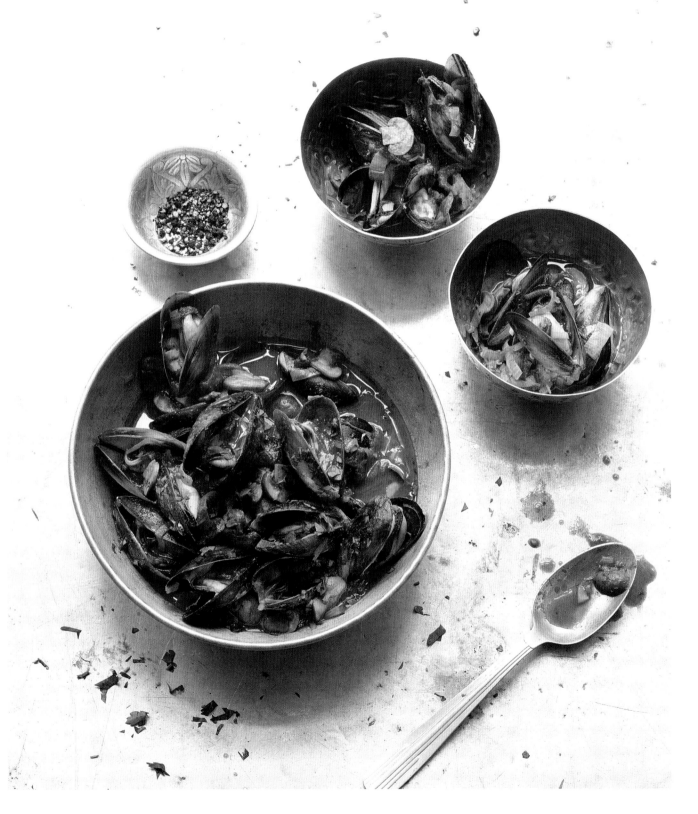

Serves 4

Ingredients

3 tbsp Moroccan Spice Rub
(see p.19)

2 small lemons, 1 sliced into thin
rings and 1 juiced

3 tbsp olive oil

1 tsp salt

4 whole red snapper fish, washed

1 white onion, peeled and
thinly sliced

½ fennel bulb, thinly sliced

2 garlic cloves, peeled and
finely chopped

10–12 sungold cherry tomatoes

a large handful of fresh coriander
(cilantro), roughly chopped

Tip

You can use either sea bass
or sea bream if you can't find
red snapper.

Tangiers Festive Fish

Ducking into the cool shady side streets of Tangier when we were
on holiday a few years ago, we noticed cars laden with flowers and
coloured boxes and trays of dried fruits being unloaded into a
beautiful courtyard. The courtyard was full of ornate mosaic tables
already laid out with blue and white dishes, red and turquoise
coloured lanterns and glasses. We followed our noses and eyes to find
that this was a family celebration and very quickly we saw a lady arrive
carrying a large oval tray with whole roasted fish stuffed with onions
and spices. Later on, we asked at our hotel about this and the owner
told us about this traditional dish that is prepared for special guests
and gave me his wife's recipe. I made it as soon as I came back and
using my Moroccan Spice Rub, this makes a delicious dish, which feels
and looks like it could be made for a celebratory meal but is quick,
simple, aromatic, wholesome and healthy.

Method

Preheat the grill to medium.

Mix 2 tablespoons Moroccan Spice Rub, 1 tablespoon lemon juice,
1 tablespoon olive oil and ½ teaspoon salt together. Score each fish
a few times across the skin on both sides. Push the mixture well into
the cuts of the fish and rub over the inside. Line the inside of each fish
with the lemon slices. Cover and chill in the refrigerator for 30 minutes.

Heat the remaining olive oil in a pan over a medium heat. Add the sliced
onions, fennel slices and garlic and cook for 3–4 minutes until soft. Add
the remaining Moroccan Spice Rub and salt, mix for 2 minutes, then add
the tomatoes and ½ tablespoon lemon juice. Check the seasoning and
add more salt if needed. Mix in the coriander leaves. Divide the fennel,
onion and tomato mixture equally between the fish and stuff into the
fish cavity.

Place the fish on a baking tray and grill on both sides until cooked. This
should take about 7–9 minutes for each side. The fish should be slightly
charred. Squeeze over a little lemon to taste before serving.

Eat with my Vine-Ripened Tomato, Sumac and Pomegranate Molasses
Salad (see p.140).

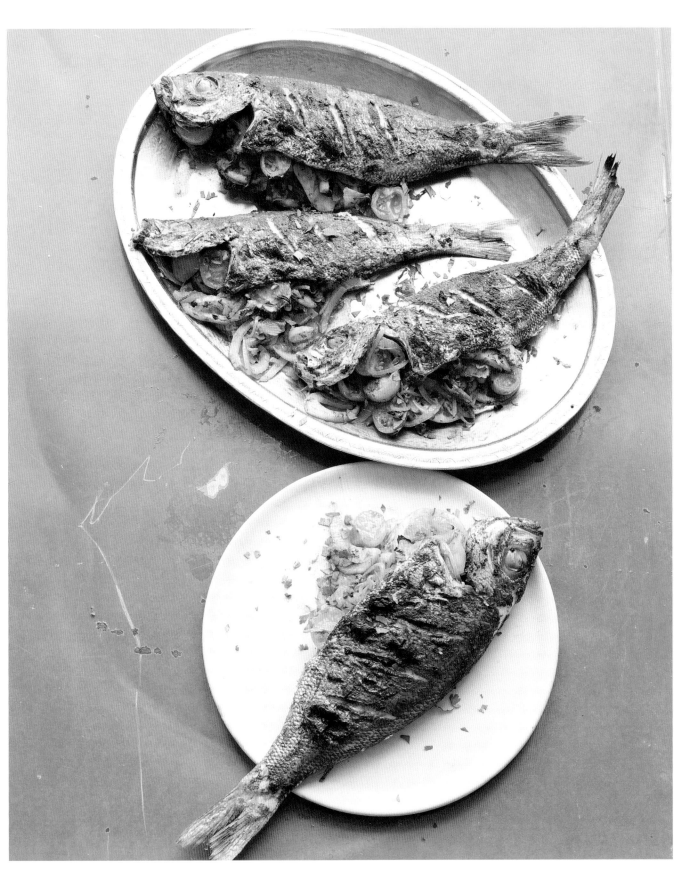

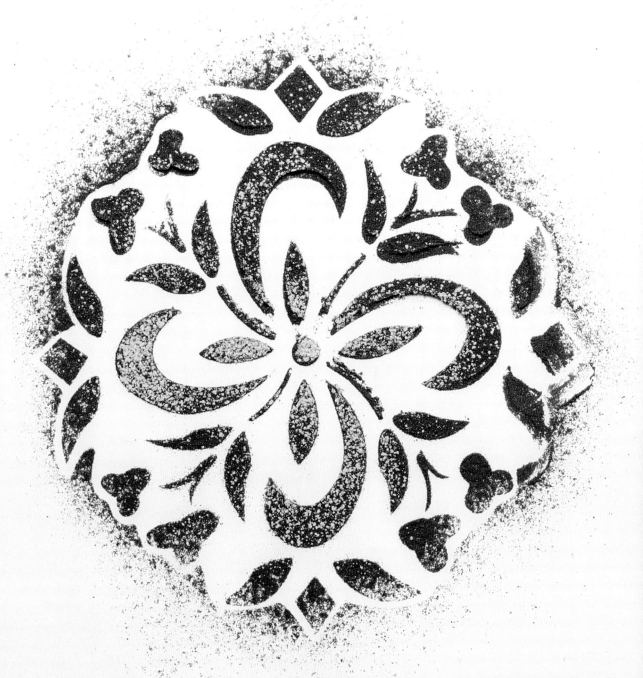

Spicetacular Sides

Side dishes are so often disregarded extras in cookery books and in meals, but for most food cultures where spices are part of the everyday cooking experience, meals often come with plentiful side dishes that are integral to adding flavour, texture, colour and different tastes to the whole eating experience. Most of the side dishes in this book can be delicious snacks or quick lunches and some can even be upscaled to main dishes in their own right. Sometimes adding a delicious side dish elevates a meal and other times, it's good to have something extra without adding too many calories.

There are in fact side dishes sprinkled throughout this book, but in this chapter you will find vibrant sides that go well with so many dishes – sweet and bright vine-ripe tomato, sumac and pomegranate molasses; and cooling protein-filled yogurt with healthy iron-rich spinach. I eat the Shaved Fennel, Fennel Seeds, Cucumber and Pomegranate Side (see p.138) as a main dish on my light eating days. It is energising and filling on its own and I often have the Beetroot and Cumin Dip (see p.142) on crackers for lunch, as it's fresh, aromatic (with the roasted cumin) and so good for you!

180 KCAL

Serves 4

Ingredients

330g/11½oz vine tomatoes, diced
½ large cucumber, peeled
   and diced
½ red onion, peeled and
   finely diced
28g/1oz fresh flat-leaf parsley,
   finely chopped
14g/½oz fresh mint leaves,
   finely chopped
1 tbsp fresh lemon juice
2 tbsp olive oil
½ tsp salt
¼ tsp freshly ground black pepper
1 large ripe avocado, peeled,
   stoned and diced
½ tbsp za'atar

My Shirazi Salad

The Persians had a great influence in India, and North India has been heavily influenced by their food, art and even language. This simple salad with its vibrant red and green colours reminds me of the beautiful colours of Moghul paintings which abound in palaces in North India. As with so many Persian and Middle Eastern dishes, fresh ingredients and herbs are key. I love this salad but often want to introduce a healthy spice, so I top it with za'atar – a lovely spice made from thyme, sumac, marjoram and sesame seeds. Each ingredient is rich in antioxidants, so together make a great healthy addition to a fresh salad.

To evoke the taste of sun-drenched days, I use vine tomatoes and creamy fresh avocado, which is loaded with potassium (more than in a banana), fibre and healthy fats. This simple salad can be eaten with a main dish for dinner or as a light lunch mixed into steamed bulgur wheat, couscous or warm pitta bread.

Method

Put the tomatoes, cucumber, onion, parsley and mint in a large bowl.

Mix the lemon juice and olive oil and salt and pepper in a small bowl and pour onto the salad. Fold in the ripe avocado and mix gently, then sprinkle over the za'atar.

Tip

Use a mixture of red and yellow tomatoes if you can get them.

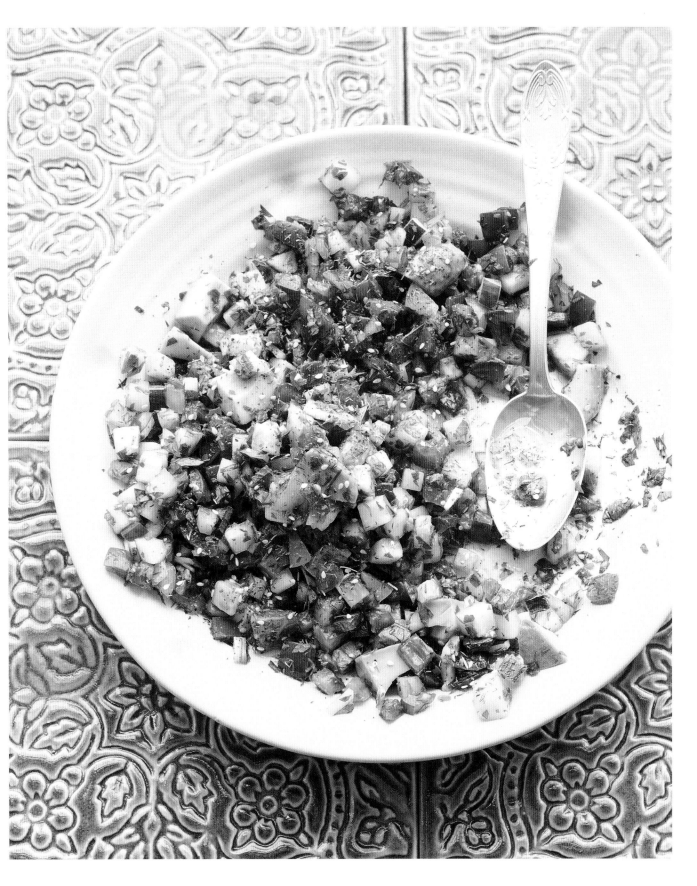

87
KCAL

Shaved Fennel, Fennel Seeds, Cucumber and Pomegranate Side

Serves 4

Ingredients

For the dressing

1 tbsp fennel seeds
1 medium eschalion shallot, peeled and finely chopped
2 tbsp good olive oil
juice of 1 small lemon
½ tsp salt
a few grinds of black pepper

For the salad

½ large cucumber
a large handful (about 25g/1oz) of rocket (arugula) leaves
1 medium fennel bulb, very thinly sliced into shavings with a mandolin or good grater
40g/1½oz fresh pomegranate seeds

This crunchy, raw and fresh salad can accompany so many dishes or be eaten on its own. This salad is spiced with nourishing fennel seeds, which are high in fibre, full of antioxidants and great for soothing digestion. Indians eat fennel with meals to aid digestion and after meals to cleanse the breath. The seeds in this dressing really give this salad a unique and refreshing taste.

Method

Dry-fry the fennel seeds so they are lightly toasted, then grind the seeds in a grinder, leaving a sprinkle whole. In a bowl or jar, mix together the rest of the dressing ingredients. Add the ground fennel seeds and mix thoroughly.

Peel the cucumber then slice in half lengthways and scoop out and discard the seeds, then cut the flesh into thin half-moon slices.

Arrange the rocket leaves in a large bowl and scatter the fennel shavings and cucumber slices on top. Pour over the dressing and mix gently. Sprinkle over the pomegranate seeds and the remaining whole fennel seeds.

Cumin and Sumac Sweet Potato Rounds

I love the simplicity and healthiness of these vegetable 'rounds' and they are so quick and easy to make. Sweet potato has so many health properties as it is a great source of antioxidants, vitamins and iron. It also has a low glycaemic index (GI) so will release energy slowly and the natural sweetness won't make your blood sugar yo-yo but will be released slowly into your bloodstream. Baking them with ancient spices – cumin and sumac – stacks up the vitamins and keeps your stomach calm and working well.

Method

Preheat the oven to 200°C/400°F/Gas mark 6.

Heat the oil in an oven dish over a medium heat and add the cumin seeds. When they start to sizzle, add the sweet potatoes and the onion and turn them in the seeds. Sprinkle with the salt and place in the hottest part of the oven for 10–12 minutes until soft. Take out of the oven and mix in the sumac, then return to the oven for about 5 minutes until the rounds are crisp. Serve immediately.

Tip

This recipe works well with butternut squash slices, carrots, parsnips, turnips and beetroots.

Serves 4

Ingredients

2 tbsp olive oil

1 tbsp cumin seeds

⅔ large sweet potato (about 400g/14oz), peeled and cut into rounds about 1cm/½in thick

1 large red onion, peeled and sliced into thin rounds

½ tsp salt

1 tbsp ground sumac

182
KCAL

Vine-Ripened Tomato, Sumac and Pomegranate Molasses

Serves 4

Ingredients

400g/14oz cherry vine-ripened
    tomatoes, cut in half
2 large vine-ripened tomatoes
    or 100g/3½oz yellow cherry
    tomatoes, cut the large
    tomatoes into small cubes and
    the cherry tomatoes in half
½ red onion, peeled
1 red or yellow (bell) pepper,
    deseeded and cut into
    thin slices
57g/2oz fresh pomegranate seeds
a small bunch of fresh coriander
    (cilantro), finely chopped
a small bunch of fresh parsley
    leaves, roughly chopped
2 small gem lettuces (about
    200g/7oz), leaves separated

For the dressing

3 tbsp extra virgin olive oil
3 tbsp pomegranate molasses
1 tsp ground sumac
¼ tsp salt

This is a lovely and colourful side dish to complement any spicy dish. Vine-ripened cherry tomatoes dressed simply with extra virgin olive oil, fragrant pomegranate molasses and zesty, beautiful ground sumac powder.

Method

Combine all the ingredients for the dressing in a bowl and whisk until mixed thoroughly.

Put all the ingredients for the salad, except the lettuce, in a bowl and pour over the dressing. Mix until the tomatoes are coated with the dressing.

Place the gem lettuce leaves on a large plate and pour the tomato salad onto the leaves.

Tip

Use the most flavourful and colourful tomatoes you can buy to really enjoy this salad.

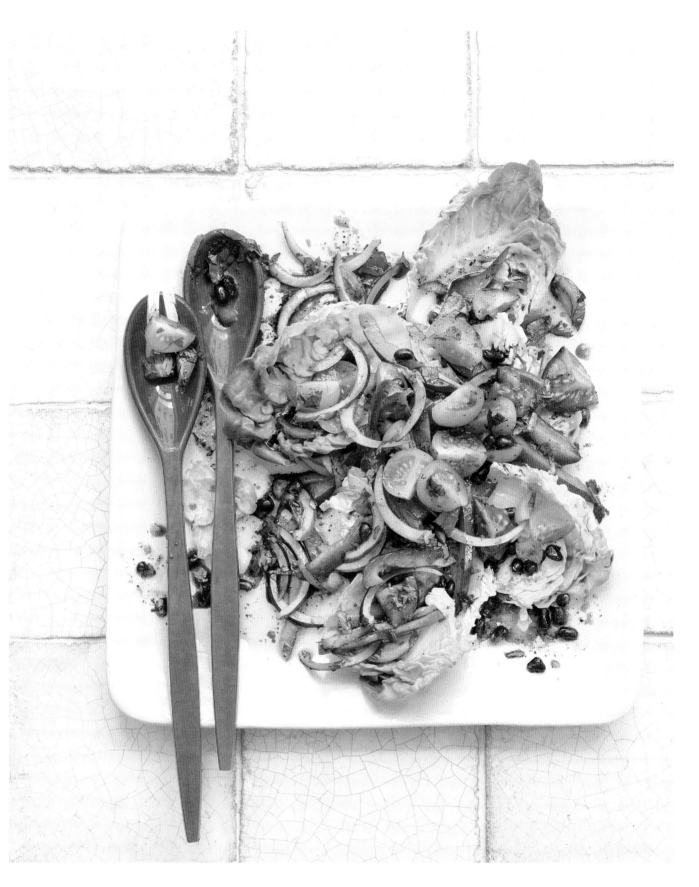

77
KCAL

Beetroot and Cumin Dip

Serves 4

Ingredients

4 medium raw beetroots
1 garlic clove
½ red chilli
2 tsp olive oil
4 tbsp lemon juice
½ tsp salt
1 tsp ground cumin
   or roast 1 tbsp cumin seeds,
   and grind (see p.167)

This is a fresh-tasting low-fat dip using just a few simple ingredients: fresh beetroot, garlic, lemon juice, salt, chilli and cumin. It is really good to eat as a snack and will keep you fuelled in between meals. It can also be eaten alongside a piece of grilled fish or chicken. The garlic is a good cleanser and the aromatic cumin will keep your digestion working well and soothed.

Method

Either bake the whole beetroots in an oven preheated to 180°C/350°F/Gas mark 4 until they are soft (this will take about 30–40 minutes) or boil the beetroots in hot water (this will take about 15–20 minutes). When soft, allow to cool then peel off the skin and grate the beetroot.

In a food processor, blend the garlic and chilli together. Mix this into the grated beetroot. Pour in the oil, lemon juice and season with the salt. Mix together and sprinkle over the ground cumin. Cover and leave in the refrigerator for 10–15 minutes before eating.

Tip

Add a spoon of plain yogurt to make this dip taste creamy.

Cool, Healthy Spinach Yogurt

55 KCAL

My family laugh at my many ways of sneaking green vegetables into everything we eat and this is one of those dishes! Spinach is so high in iron and a 'superfood', and I will eat it with most dishes I prepare. Garlic, ground cumin and fresh herbs combined with protein-rich plain yogurt make this dish nutritious and tasty!

Method

Blanch the spinach leaves in hot water then quickly plunge them into a bowl of cold water. Strain, drain well and squeeze out any excess water. Chop finely and set aside.

Mash the garlic with the salt and set aside.

Put the yogurt into a large bowl and mix in the garlic paste. Add the drained spinach and the remaining ingredients, then leave to stand for 5–10 minutes to let everything mix together. Sprinkle over the ground cumin.

Serves 4

Ingredients

100g/3½oz baby spinach leaves
2 garlic cloves, peeled and very finely chopped
½ tsp salt
300g/10½oz /1¼ cups plain yogurt
1 tbsp lemon juice
4 spring onions (scallions), finely chopped
10–12 fresh mint leaves
a large handful of fresh coriander (cilantro) leaves
½–1 tsp ground cumin

Cucumber and Mint Raita

49 KCAL

This is a classic cooling dip and accompaniment to so many dishes including kebabs, patties, roast meats, etc. I roast and grind cumin seeds to sprinkle on this raita for a burst of fragrance and health.

Method

Heat a small frying pan over a medium heat. Add the cumin seeds and roast for 2–3 minutes. Grind to a powder, then set aside.

Mix all the ingredients, except the ground cumin, together in a bowl then sprinkle the cumin over the top just before serving.

Tips

- For a special dinner – sprinkle pomegranate seeds on top.
- If grating the cucumber, squeeze out excess liquid before adding to the yogurt.

Serves 4

Ingredients

1 tbsp cumin seeds
½ large cucumber, peeled and finely chopped or grated
½ onion, peeled and very finely chopped
250g/9oz/generous 1 cup plain yogurt
a small handful of fresh mint leaves, finely chopped
a small handful of fresh coriander (cilantro) leaves, finely chopped
1 tsp lemon juice
¼ tsp salt

Ginger and Cardamom Snack Jack

Makes 20 squares

Ingredients

85g/3oz/1 cup rolled oats
30g/1oz/scant ¼ cup hazelnuts, roughly chopped or bashed in a tea towel with a rolling pin
1 tbsp flaxseeds, milled
75g/2½oz/⅔ cup toasted pumpkin and sunflower seeds
50g/1¾oz//⅓ cup dried raisins and dried cranberries, roughly chopped
1 tsp dried ginger
5cm/2in piece fresh ginger, peeled and finely grated
¾ tsp ground cardamom powder
2 tbsp rapeseed (canola) oil
3 tbsp runny honey
2 tbsp warm water

This is healthy and filling snack that will keep you going in between meals. It's good to have a few healthy (but tasty) snacks around when you feel hungry or are craving something sweet. This 'snack jack' is full of good ingredients including oats (filling and good for your heart), hazelnuts (full of protein), fresh ginger (great for warding off colds), ground cardamom powder (an aromatic spice which soothes digestion) and honey to add a natural sweetness.

Method

Preheat the oven to 150°C/300°F/Gas mark 2 and line a baking tray with greaseproof paper.

Mix all the dry ingredients together into a bowl. Pour in the oil, honey and warm water and mix thoroughly.

Place the mixture on the baking tray and smooth with a palette knife. Press it down to make it even. Bake in the oven for 16–18 minutes.

Take it out of the oven and allow to cool, then cut into squares.

Tips
- Make a batch and it will keep in an airtight container for 5–6 days.
- Cut it into small pieces so you limit yourself to one piece at a time.
- You can buy ready-ground cardamom powder or you can make it yourself by bashing 6–8 cardamom pods with a pestle, taking out the seeds and grinding in a mortar into a very fine powder.

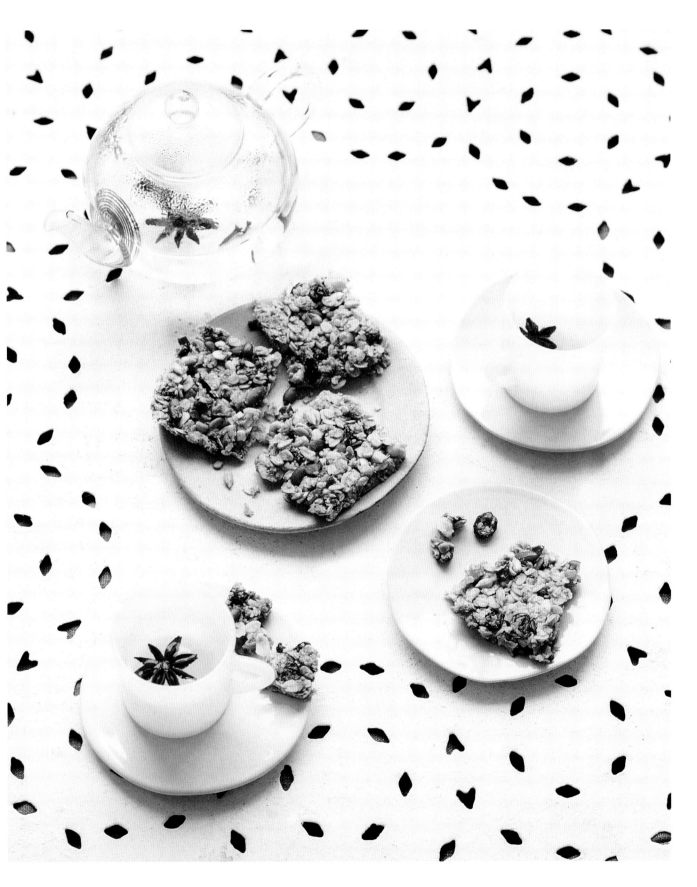

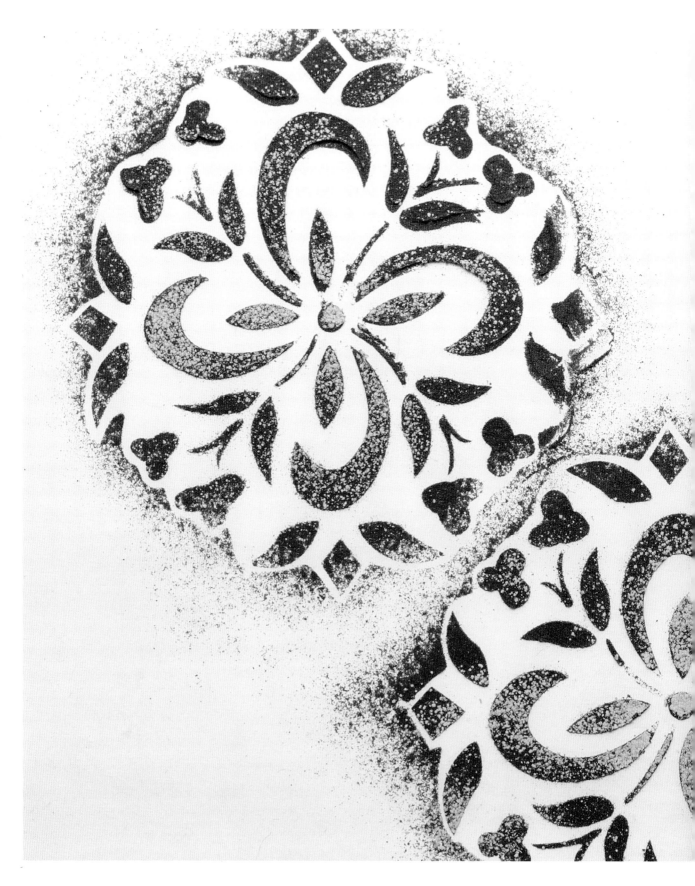

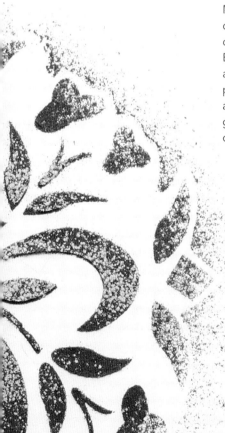

Tantalising Sweet Treats

Most diet books either ban desserts altogether or suggest such dull options that they don't feel like much of a treat at all. No one said you can't have sweet treats and they don't all have to be full of fat and calories. By using some everyday fruits such as strawberries, bananas and peaches alongside some of their more exotic cousins such as mango, star fruit and passion fruit (all of which are now regular fixtures in most supermarket fruit aisles) and then combining them with spices as diverse as cardamom, chilli, ginger and cinnamon, you can create some really wonderful and enjoyable desserts that are refreshingly different and also healthy.

162
KCAL

Saffron Mango and Passion Fruit Shrikhand

Serves 4

Ingredients

200g/7oz/generous ¾ cup whole
Greek yogurt
200g/7oz/generous ¾ cup low-fat
Greek yogurt
½ tbsp soft light brown sugar
½ tsp ground cardamom powder
made from 6 small
cardamom pods
a pinch of red chilli (red pepper)
flakes (optional)
5–6 saffron threads
3 tbsp semi-skimmed (low-fat)
milk, warmed
1 large mango, peeled, stoned
and cut into small cubes
1 passion fruit, cut in half and
seeds spooned out
a small handful of roasted flaked
(slivered) almonds
a small handful of redcurrants and
raspberries (optional)

Shrikhand is an Indian dessert usually made from yogurt that is hung in a muslin cloth for about 4–5 hours until all the whey drains away and you are left with the creamy solids. I love shrikhand but I don't have the time always to wait, so I make it with a mixture of low-fat and whole creamy Greek yogurt. As in most Indian desserts, warm spices are added to enhance the flavour and to increase the health benefits. Saffron and cardamom are the spices in this dessert and both will help with digestion. I have also added a sneaky pinch of chilli – I love the slight kick it gives this dessert!

Method

In a large bowl, whisk together both the yogurts with the brown sugar until creamy. Stir in the ground cardamom powder and chilli flakes and set aside.

In another bowl, soak the saffron strands in the warm milk for a few minutes. When the colour of the milk turns a lovely light orange, strain and add the milk to the yogurt and sugar mixture.

Gently fold in the mango and passion fruit, then scoop the mixture into 4 small bowls and chill in the refrigerator for at least 1 hour. When serving, sprinkle each dish with a few flaked almonds and top with the redcurrants and raspberries (if using).

Tips

- You can use any fruit you like – pineapples or strawberries work well. I like to top the dessert with fresh redcurrants and raspberries.
- To make the ground cardamom powder – just bash the cardamom pods with a pestle, take out the seeds and grind them in a mortar into a very fine powder.

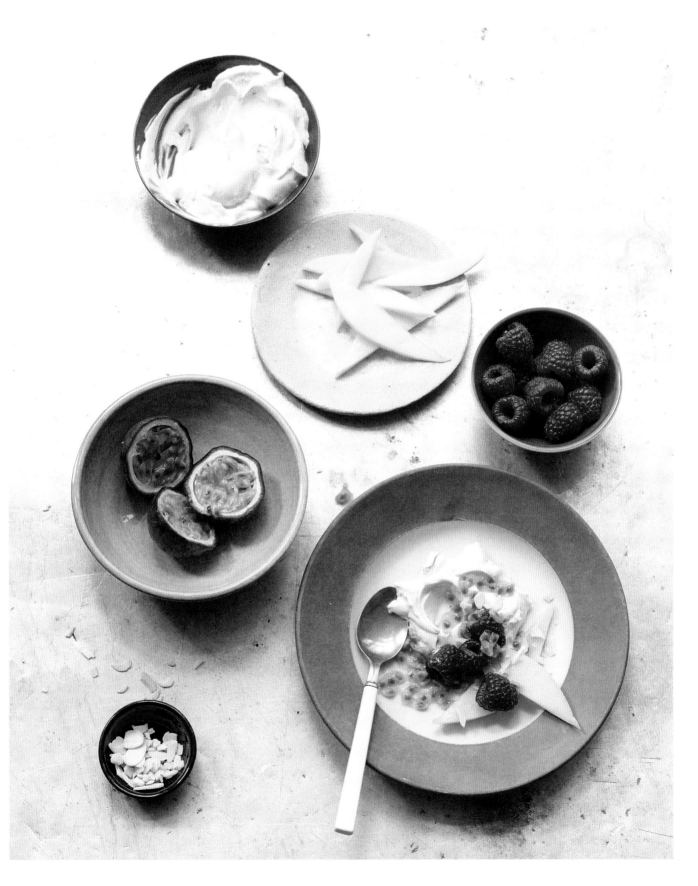

Warming Fruity Oat Crumble

A guilt-free and gluten-free dessert, this is a hearty pudding with just a light covering of oaty crumble. You can use any fruit depending on the season. I love crumble in the winter, and when rhubarb is available I like to include it as it adds a lovely tart flavour. To balance the tartness I use cinnamon – a natural sweetener and packed with goodness, as well as maple syrup which adds a toffee-like sweetness (make sure it's not maple-flavoured syrup as this is not genuine and often has other sugars added to it). To make this dessert super-healthy and warming, I add ginger to keep those winter bugs at bay and to help keep joints moving as it has tremendous anti-inflammatory properties. Ginger also helps digest the fruit sugars in the dessert and the cinnamon will keep your sugar levels steady to stop too many sugar cravings.

Serves 4

Ingredients

2 Bramley or cooking apples, cored and cut into cubes
5cm/2in piece fresh ginger, peeled and finely grated
2 tbsp maple syrup
2 tbsp fresh orange juice
1 cinnamon stick
100ml/3½fl oz/scant ½ cup warm water
1 large rhubarb stalk, cut into large cubes

For the crumble topping

56g/2oz/4 tbsp organic butter, at room temperature
100g/3½oz/1¼ cups rolled oats
¾ tsp ground cinnamon

Method

Preheat the oven to 200°C/400°F/Gas mark 6.

Place the apple pieces, ginger, 1 tablespoon maple syrup, orange juice and the cinnamon stick (and star anise, if using) in a large pan with the water and gently cook on a medium-low heat for 5 minutes. Add the rhubarb pieces and cook until almost soft.

In a bowl, crumble the butter into the oats with your fingertips. Sprinkle the cinnamon over this mixture.

Put the cooked fruit, including cinnamon stick, into a baking dish and sprinkle the crumble mixture over the top. Drizzle the remaining maple syrup over the topping and bake in the hot oven for 15–20 minutes. Serve hot with a spoonful of plain yogurt.

Tip

Add 2 star anise with the cinnamon stick to give the filling extra flavour.

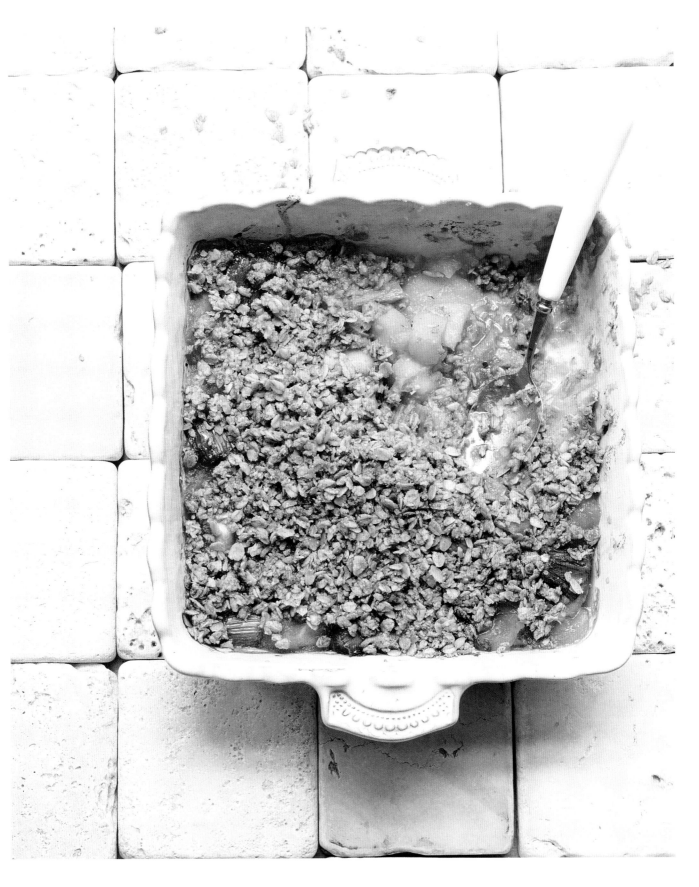

Sticky and Spicy Pineapple and Banana with Cinnamon

Serves 4

Ingredients

2 bananas
5 tbsp lemon juice
½ pineapple, peeled and cored and cut into wedges (you will need 4–6 wedges per person)
1 tbsp ground cinnamon
3 tbsp runny honey
2 tbsp toasted sesame seeds
6 tbsp plain yogurt
8–10 fresh mint leaves

This is a very quick and simple dessert. I love sticky bananas and this reminds me of banana fritters without the frying! A sweet treat without sugar but with healthy honey and cinnamon instead. The cinnamon adds natural sweetness with no extra calories and I find that honey doesn't make me crave sugary things – it has a satisfying sweetness but adds a stickiness which makes the fruit all the more delicious!

Method

Preheat the grill to high.

Peel the bananas and slice down the middle and then in half. Put the bananas in a bowl and mix in the lemon juice (this will stop them from going brown). Place the pineapple wedges in a separate bowl, then sprinkle the bananas with half the ground cinnamon and the pineapple with the other half.

Place the fruit (reserve the lemon juice from the bananas) on a foil-lined grill pan and cook for 2–3 minutes or until starting to colour. Quickly remove the fruit from the grill.

In a large non-stick sauté pan, gently heat the honey and lemon juice and, when warm, add the sesame seeds. Carefully add the pineapple and bananas and gently toss in the mixture. The fruit should be coated and when the honey begins to stick, take them out of the pan and serve immediately topped with the yogurt and mint leaves.

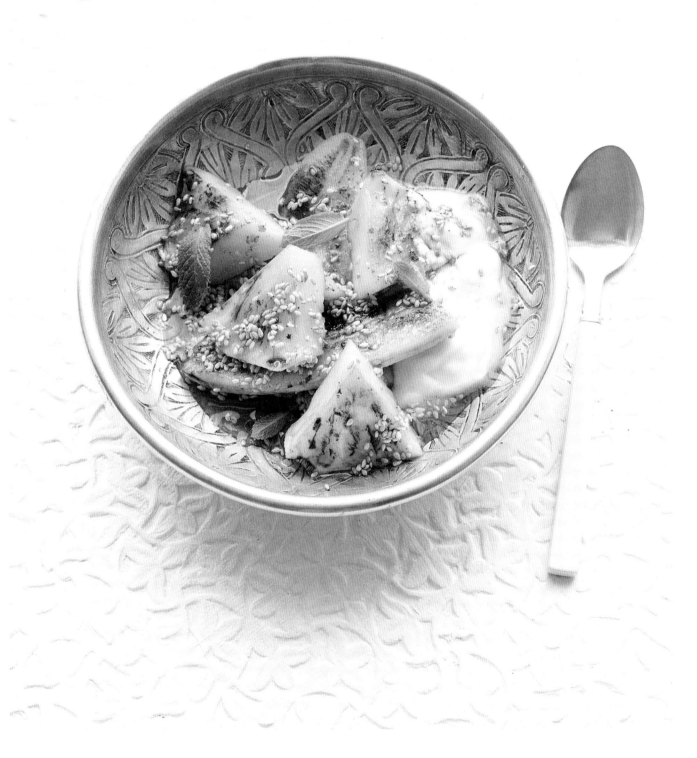

Rose Water Scented Rhubarb and Strawberries

Serves 4

Ingredients

For the vanilla yogurt

1 vanilla pod (bean)
200g/7oz/generous ¾ cup plain live yogurt

For the rhubarb and strawberries

300g/10½oz rhubarb stalks, trimmed and cut into 2.5cm/1in strips
1–2 tbsp rose water (see tips below)
5cm/2in piece fresh ginger, peeled and roughly sliced
½ tsp ground ginger
4 tbsp warm water
¼ tsp ground cardamom powder made from grinding the seeds from 4 pods
2 tbsp demerara (raw brown) sugar
200g/7oz/scant 1½ cups strawberries, sliced

I love the rosy pink and tangy sweetness of rhubarb teamed with red strawberries, and both these fruits go very well with spices. To easily digest the acidity of the rhubarb and strawberries, I add a small measure of fresh and dried ginger (dried ginger has a sharper taste than fresh) and a sprinkle of ground cardamom seeds. To elevate the dish to dizzy heights, I add a judicious few drops of rose water – beautiful, aromatic and heady! I love it. Serve hot or cool with vanilla-infused plain yogurt for a delicious dessert or eat with your porridge or granola for a yummy breakfast.

Method

Preheat the oven to 180°C/350°F/Gas mark 4.

Start by making the vanilla yogurt. Slice the vanilla pod down the middle and scrape out the seeds. Mix the seeds into the plain yogurt and leave to infuse for 20–30 minutes while cooking the fruit.

Place a large piece of foil paper (large enough to make a parcel with the rhubarb and strawberries) in a deep baking tray and add the rhubarb. Sprinkle the rose water, fresh and dried ginger, warm water, ground cardamom powder and sugar over the rhubarb, then fold over to make a parcel. Bake in the hot oven for 12–15 minutes, or when the rhubarb is almost soft. Carefully open the parcel and add the strawberries. Cover and continue baking for a further 5 minutes until the strawberries and rhubarb are soft.

Remove the ginger and mix the fruit and juices together gently. Divide the fruit into 4 servings. Top the fruit with equal amounts of the yogurt and spoon over some of the juice.

Tips

- If you have never cooked with rose water, start with 1 tablespoon. If you can't find it in the shops, you can use a vanilla pod, split lengthways in half, and add this to the dish when baking the rhubarb.
- For the ground cardamom powder, bash the pods with a pestle, take out the seeds and grind in the mortar into a very fine powder.
- If you are entertaining, then top with a few mint leaves or an edible rose petal on each serving to make it look beautiful.

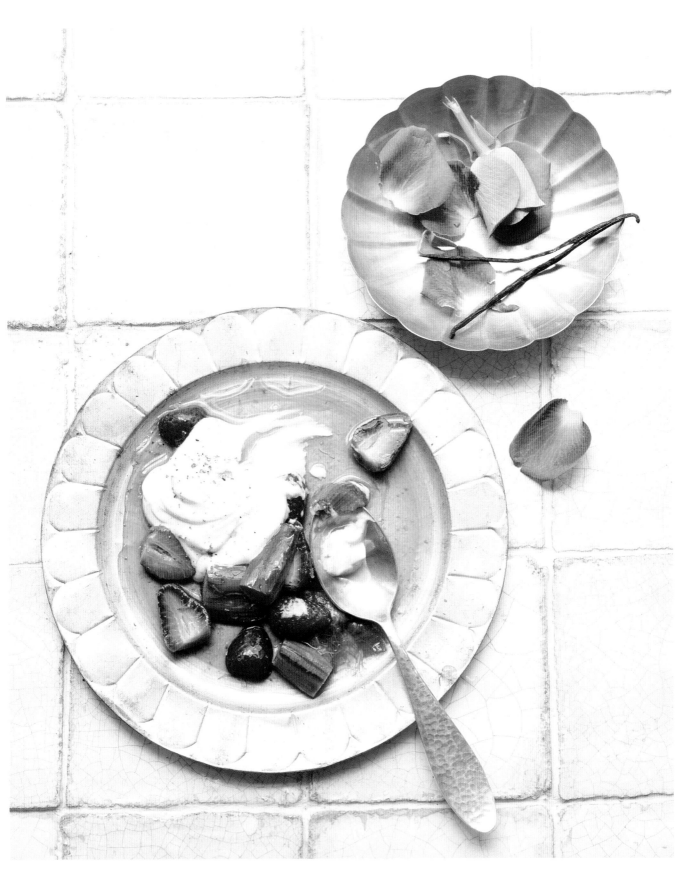

213
KCAL

Mango, Chilli and Black Pepper Mess

Serves 4

Ingredients

500g/1lb 2oz/2¼ cups zero-fat
   Greek yogurt, stirred well
1 tbsp muscovado (brown) sugar
1 star anise
1 tsp vanilla extract
1 large ripe mango, peeled,
   stoned and cut into cubes
200g/7oz/scant 1½ cups fresh
   strawberries, sliced,
   save 4 whole strawberries
   for the topping
½ tablespoon fresh lime juice
½ tsp chilli powder
freshly ground black pepper
3 tbsp chopped nuts, such as
   walnuts or pecans
a small handful of fresh mint
   leaves, save a few sprigs
   to decorate

In India, as the fruit is so sweet, it is normal to sprinkle black pepper (just a few grinds) and sometimes chilli over mango to add a spicy edge. Don't be put off – this is a sweet dish with a 'warm' undertone. The chilli gives the mango a small kick, lifts the taste and adds a big kick of health benefits as well. The Greek yogurt is infused with star anise to give it a lovely sweet, luscious taste and helps with digestion.

Method

In a bowl, gently mix the Greek yogurt with the sugar until smooth. Stir in the star anise and vanilla extract, then cover and leave to infuse for 30 minutes.

In a separate bowl, combine the mango and strawberries then sprinkle over the lime juice, chilli, mint leaves and black pepper. Mix gently and set aside.

Remove the star anise from the yogurt. Layer the fruit mixture into 4 small glasses (high ball) followed by the yogurt. Top with nuts, a strawberry and a sprig of mint.

Tip

I like to add a bit of crunch (and protein) by topping the desserts with finely chopped walnuts or pecans.

Kim's Pear and Ginger Gluten-Free Crumble

(using stevia) (using sugar)

Kim Ingleby is probably the most healthy, wonderful person I know. A multi-award-winning personal trainer, she has mentored me through the years in fitness, mental strength, health and well-being. This is her healthy dessert recipe. It is gluten free and includes lovely spices, which will make you feel great and do you good too. Traditional Chinese five-spice is a heady mix of spices including Szechuan pepper, fennel, cinnamon, cloves and beautiful star anise. It sometimes includes ginger and other warming spices. All these spices have powerful health benefits, soothing the digestion and helping to regulate blood sugar levels. Gluten-free flour works as well as normal flour. Stevia is a naturally sourced sugar from the Stevia plant, which grows in Brazil and Paraguay. It is low in carbohydrate and calorie free, but it is very sweet, so adjust the amount according to taste.

Method

Preheat the oven to 200°C/400°F/Gas mark 6.

To make the filling, boil the water. Add the chopped pears, ginger, lime zest and juice, and simmer for 5–8 minutes until the pears are softened.

Meanwhile, sift the flour into a bowl and add the spices and sugar. Cut the butter into small cubes and rub it into the flour with your fingertips until it resembles fine breadcrumbs. Mix in the rolled oats.

Place the cooked pear mixture into a baking dish and sprinkle the crumble evenly over the top. Bake in the hot oven for 20 minutes. Sprinkle the flaked almonds, chia seeds and salt over the top then bake for a further 5 minutes. Take out of the oven, serve and enjoy!

Serves 4

Ingredients

For the topping

120g/4oz/1 cup gluten-free flour mix
1 tsp Chinese five-spice powder
45g/1½oz/¼cup unrefined brown sugar or stevia
60g/2oz/4 tbsp butter or coconut butter, softened
50g/1¾oz/½ cup rolled oats
50g/1¾oz/½ cup flaked (slivered) almonds
chia seeds and pink sea salt, for topping

For the filling

100ml/3½fl oz/scant ½ cup water
3–4 pears, peeled, chopped and deseeded
30g/1oz piece fresh ginger, peeled and grated
finely grated zest and juice of 1 lime

Good-For-You Chocolate and Cardamom Pots

Serves 4

Ingredients

75g/2½oz dark chocolate, broken into small cubes
1 tsp organic cocoa powder, plus ½ tbsp for dusting
½ tsp vanilla extract
½ tsp ground cardamom powder
60g/2¼oz/¼ cup low-fat fromage frais
2 egg whites
1 tbsp caster (superfine) sugar
150g/5¼oz/1 cup strawberries, thinly sliced

Tips

- Always use dark chocolate with at least 70–80% cocoa solids.
- I love to top these pots with strawberries but blueberries or raspberries are good too.
- To make the ground cardamom powder – just bash the cardamom pods with a pestle, take out the seeds and grind them in a mortar into a very fine powder.

Good for you? Well, good chocolate with high cocoa solids is good for you as it is rich in antioxidants and, I don't know about you, but anything with good chocolate always makes me smile and feel great. Add the warming powder made from the seeds from the cardamom pod and you have an intriguing shot of flavour and also a shot of nutrition. Cardamom is related to ginger and has some of the same health benefits. It helps with digestion, soothes bloating and cleanses the body. Note: with cardamom, less is more, so you only need to add a little of this sumptuous spice.

Method

Place a heatproof bowl over a pan of simmering (not boiling) water. Add the chocolate, cocoa powder, vanilla extract and ground cardamom powder and slowly melt. When melted, take off the heat and allow to cool.

Mix the fromage frais gently into the cooled chocolate mixture until everything is combined.

Whisk the egg whites in a freestanding electric mixer until stiff, then slowly add the sugar while still beating. You should have glossy peaks. Slowly fold half the egg white mixture into the chocolate mixture until it is mixed in, then add the rest and fold in gently. Don't beat the mixture – the trick is to keep it light and airy.

Place a few strawberry slices at the base of each ramekin or espresso cup and put a portion of the chocolate mixture into each pot. Top with more strawberries. Chill in the refrigerator for around 45 minutes until set.

Dust each pot with the remaining cocoa powder before serving.

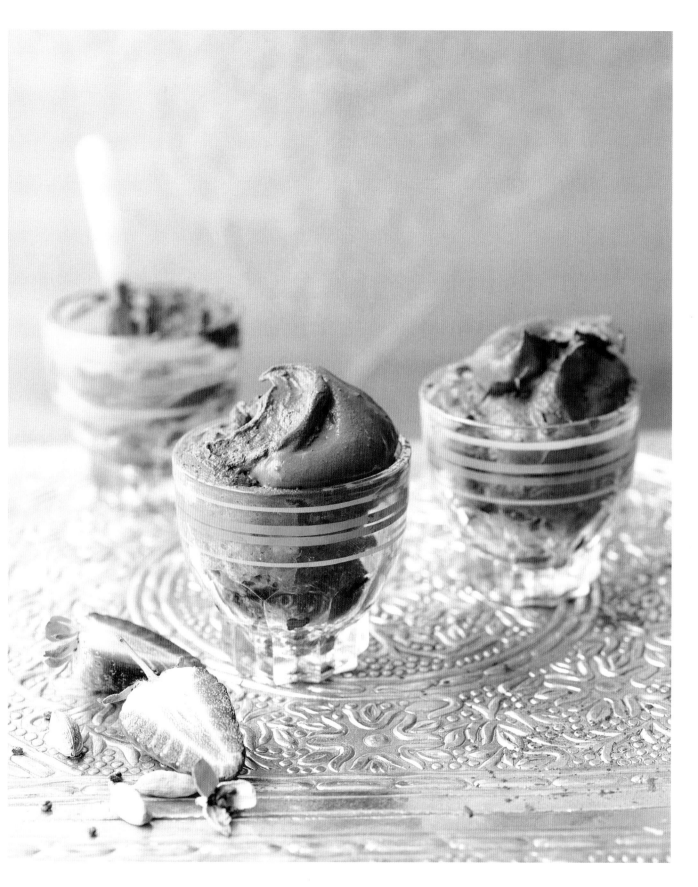

179
KCAL

Cardamom and Star Anise Baked Peaches

Serves 4

Ingredients

4 ripe peaches, halved and stoned
3 tbsp runny honey
4 tbsp warm water
28g/1oz/2 tbsp butter
1 star anise
5–6 green cardamom pods, smashed lightly so that the seeds can infuse the dish
a small handful of flaked (slivered) almonds
4 tbsp plain yogurt

Fruit can take time to digest and adding the right spices helps this process. This is a simple, slow-baked dessert with aromatic cardamom, which will soothe your digestion at the end of a meal. Star anise is a gorgeous star-shaped fruit with a unique, deep liquorice flavour and has been traditionally used to relieve stomach pain and digestive problems. This dessert is definitely satisfying and healthy.

Method

Preheat the oven to 180°C/350°F/Gas mark 4.

Place the peaches face down in an ovenproof bowl.

Mix together the honey and water and pour over the peaches. Crumble over the butter, then add the star anise and cardamom pods. Bake in the hot oven for 10–15 minutes until the peaches are soft and the juices are mixed in. Discard the star anise before serving. Turn the peaches so they are facing up, sprinkle over the flaked almonds, and serve topped with the plain yogurt.

Tips

• You can use peaches, apricots or nectarines for this dish.
• When cool, it can be kept in the refrigerator and then eaten cold.
• A light sprinkling of rose water before the peaches go into the oven will really make this dessert feel special.

Baked Pears
with Walnut Cream

Pears and walnuts go together so well – in a salad as well as a dessert. This is a simple dish with all the goodness of the hot fruit, sweetened with cinnamon, spicy cloves, lush honey, and a cold cream made from chopped walnuts and ricotta cheese.

Method

Preheat the oven to 180°C/350°F/Gas mark 4.

Mix the ricotta, cinnamon, 1 tablespoon of the runny honey, lime zest and lime juice together in a bowl until smooth. Mix in the crushed walnuts and set aside.

Prepare the pears by peeling and slice in half. Scoop out the core and make a hollow in the centre of each half. Place the water and cloves in a non-stick baking dish and place the pears face down in the dish. Drizzle the remaining honey over the pears and cover with foil.

Bake in the hot oven for 15–20 minutes until the pears are soft. Take out of the oven, turn the pear halves over, and divide the ricotta and walnut cream between them. Return to the oven for 5 minutes.

After 5 minutes, spoon over any honey left in the baking dish (discard the cloves) and dust with a sprinkling of cinnamon before serving.

Serves 4

Ingredients

70g/2½oz/⅓ cup soft ricotta cheese
1 tsp ground cinnamon, plus a little extra for dusting
3 tbsp runny honey
zest and juice of ½ small lime
8–10 walnut halves, roughly chopped
2 eating pears
100ml/3½fl oz/scant ½ cup warm water
4–6 cloves

Drinks To Spice Yourself Slim

These are cleansing drinks and ones that will help you keep nourished and your digestion calm through the day. With the exception of Golden Tea, they are all zero calories.

Ginger is very good in the morning as it helps to detoxify the body. Cinnamon is good in the afternoon if you're flagging as it is naturally sweet and doesn't play havoc with your glucose levels. Fennel is a cleanser and a good digestive, while cayenne pepper can help to shift the metabolism into working better and cloves can protect the immune system so will keep bugs at bay.

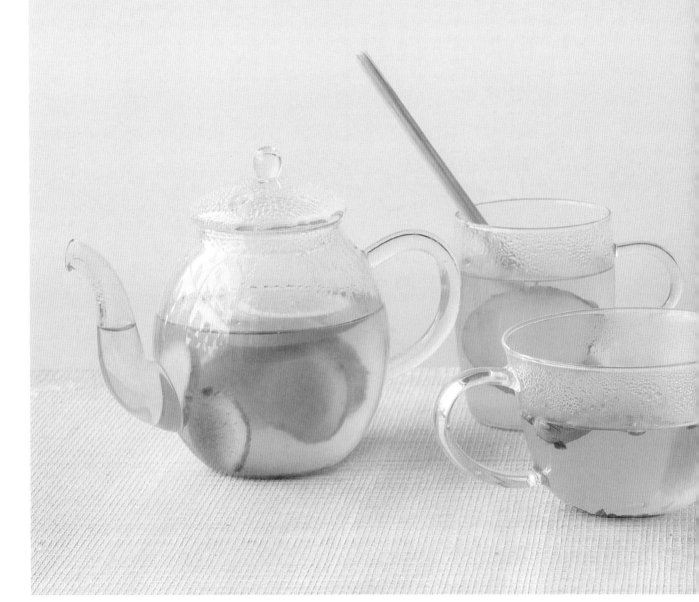

1 Fennel and Ginger

Add 1 piece of fresh ginger, peeled and grated, to a heatproof glass with 1 teaspoon fennel seeds and pour over freshly boiled water. Allow to steep for 4–5 minutes. Strain and drink while the water is warm.

2 Ginger and Lemon

Add 1 piece fresh ginger, peeled and grated, to a heatproof glass with a large slice of lemon. Pour over freshly boiled water and allow to steep for 4–5 minutes. Strain and drink while the water is warm.

3 Ginger, Lemon and Cayenne Pepper

Add 1 piece of fresh ginger, peeled and grated, to a heatproof glass with ¼ teaspoon cayenne powder. Pour over freshly boiled water and allow to steep for 4–5 minutes. Strain and drink while the water is warm.

4 Star Anise and Clove

Add 1 star anise and 3–4 cloves to a heatproof glass of freshly boiled water. Allow to cool, then remove the star anise and cloves, and drink with a dash of honey.

5 Cinnamon and Cloves

Add 1 cinnamon stick and 3–4 cloves to a heatproof glass of freshly boiled water. Allow to cool, then remove the cinnamon stick and cloves, and drink with a dash of honey.

6 Cardamom and Fennel

Smash 2–3 cardamom pods a little, then add to a heatproof glass of freshly boiled water. Add ½ teaspoon fennel seeds and mint, if you like, then strain before drinking.

7 Lemongrass, Ginger and Basil

Add 2.5cm/1in piece of fresh ginger, peeled and grated, to a heatproof glass. Bruise ½ lemongrass stalk by giving it a bash, then add it to the glass with some fresh basil. Pour on freshly boiled water and allow to infuse for 5 minutes. Drink while still warm.

8 Turmeric, Ginger and Lemon

Add 1 piece of fresh ginger, peeled and grated, to a heatproof glass of freshly boiled water. Mix in ¼ teaspoon ground turmeric and a slice of lemon, and add a dash of honey, if required.

9 Golden Tea (aka Golden Milk)
19 calories

Serves 2, makes 200ml/7fl oz/scant 1 cup.
Simply grind 13g/½oz grated turmeric root or ¾ teaspoon ground turmeric and 2.5cm/1in piece fresh ginger, peeled and grated, with ½ teaspoon coconut oil in a pestle and mortar to make a smooth paste. Mix in ¼ teaspoon freshly ground black pepper. Warm 200ml/7fl oz/scant 1 cup coconut or almond milk over a low heat, then stir in the ginger paste and stir slowly until the milk is nearly boiling (don't bring it to the boil). Turn off the heat and allow to steep for 3–4 minutes. Strain through a tea strainer and stir in ¼ teaspoon honey, if you like. Drink while warm.

Spice Directory

Buying Spices

As with anything – you get what you pay for. Go for organic and from a reputable supplier and buy in small quantities unless you are making a batch of spice mix. Spices lose their goodness and taste horrible if they are kept for too long.

Buying whole spices versus buying ground spices

The process of roasting whole spices and grinding them by hand evokes nostalgic memories for me, but it is also the best way to make the most of spices. Roasting whole seeds and spices releases their aroma and oils, and, I think, elevates and intensifies the taste of the spice. Freshly roasted and ground cumin has an intense flavour, which isn't fully replicated in the powder. This is the same for coriander seeds and Szechuan pepper. Some spices are very hard to grind by hand, such as cinnamon sticks and black cardamoms, so I often use an electric grinder, which is quick, easy and doesn't alter the taste.

The flavour of whole spices and ground can sometimes differ. Whole coriander seeds have a more citrusy flavour than ground coriander, and ground cumin isn't hugely aromatic unless roasted. However, good ground powders are available and they can be used in most recipes unless the recipe specifically calls for the whole seed to be used.

Fresh ginger has a lively, edgy taste while the dried variety tastes very different and is almost sweet, bitter and spicy. Fresh garlic has a lively fragrance but dried garlic often has a dull fragrance and not as much bite as fresh.

Taking Care of Your Spices

Spices mean so much to me I take care of them. I want their taste, colour, freshness and goodness to be at their peak when I use them. Spices lose their taste, aroma and goodness over time, so I don't keep any spices for more than six months. It is best to keep them in a cool, dry cupboard away from sunlight and in airtight containers (oxygen will erode the taste and quality). It is also good to keep them away from the heat and steam of cooking, as you don't want air or moisture getting into the container.

Our family, and most Indians, keep their main spices in a masala dhaba or tin. It is a steel tin with a tight-fitting lid and has up to seven pots inside. Some also come with little spoons for each spice. The choice of spices comes from the most often used, so in my own tin I have turmeric, chilli powder, cumin seeds, ground coriander, garam masala and a bowl of whole spices (cassia bark, cloves, peppercorns and dried bay leaves) which I like to use with pilaus and some meats. However, the pots in the tin are not labelled, so unless you are familiar with your spices, I recommend using glass jars and advise you to label each jar with the name of the spice and the date.

Key Spices

The recipes in this book require ten main storecupboard spices:

- Turmeric
- Chilli
- Cumin seeds
- Cinnamon and cinnamon bark
- Coriander seeds and ground coriander
- Cloves
- Cardamom
- Fennel seeds
- Carom seeds
- Fenugreek seeds

In addition, I have included two familiar fresh spices:

- Garlic
- Ginger

You will also find four exciting new spices that have been introduced to us by chefs from around the world. These are:

- Sumac
- Saffron (not new to us but we are using this more now)
- Star anise
- Szechuan peppers

Finally, I have added two more delightful and exotic spice mixes:

- Ras el hanout
- Za'atar

Fresh Spices for Everyday Health

Garlic
Fresh garlic is an amazing spice and it packs huge health benefits. I use it in a lot of recipes because it contains a compound called allicin, which protects cells and supports and helps to strengthen the immune system. In fact, its use as a health spice dates back 5,000 years. Not only did the ancient Egyptians and Greeks believe that garlic is powerful in fighting off sickness, but throughout the centuries the Chinese, Indians and other cultures from around the world have been using garlic as a medicinal spice to stave off illness. It's very good for digestion and my family have used it for years to help cleanse the body, as it's also a great detoxifier. My father would say that garlic cleanses the blood. Studies are now showing that garlic helps to maintain the respiratory and blood circulation systems in our bodies. Garlic is also rich in vitamin C and high in antioxidants and potassium. It also has antiseptic properties and was used to fight infection and gangrene in World Wars I and II.

Ginger
Fresh ginger is a root and belongs to the same plant family as turmeric and cardamom. It has been cultivated all over the world and records show its use as a medicine and a culinary spice for centuries.

Fresh ginger is one spice that I recommend keeping on hand in your kitchen at all times. Not only is it a wonderful addition to your cooking, but it also has enormous health benefits. In the world of spices, ginger has to be crowned number one in supporting the digestive system. It has long been used in India and China to help treat stomach upsets and nausea. A cup of hot water with crushed ginger and honey is a usual remedy for these conditions. However, science is now showing that ginger is a powerful anti-inflammatory, which means that it helps to alleviate pain in illnesses such as arthritis, which is caused by inflammation of the joints. Its properties also prevent illnesses occurring. Ginger has a warming, or thermogenic, effect on the body, which means that it can boost the metabolism. Drinking a glass of warm water infused with sliced ginger is a great way of keeping healthy and keeping bugs away.

Fresh ginger has a strong taste but this mellows with cooking, giving a lovely edge to any dish. Fresh ginger is used in Asian savoury dishes but dried ginger is very different and quite acerbic, so doesn't really work as a substitute to fresh ginger in Asian dishes. It generally works well in sweet dishes like cakes and breads. Pickled ginger is largely used in Japanese food.

Turmeric
In the spice jungle turmeric is the king! It has been acclaimed through history as an antiseptic, keeping

the body free from illness and bugs, and it has been used as a preventative as well as to treat illness. It is high in antioxidants and is an anti-inflammatory, so can keep your body functioning, helping it to heal quickly as well as fighting illness. New scientific research has shown that the compound in turmeric – curcumin – is a potential treatment for dementia.

Turmeric has been used in India for thousands of years as both a culinary and medicinal spice. It is also known as 'Indian saffron' but it doesn't have the delicate taste or lightness of saffron. Most of the world's turmeric comes from, and is consumed in, India. It is an orange-coloured root (fresh turmeric looks like fresh ginger), which is available now in shops, but it is normally used as a powder. Turmeric provides the yellow colour in curries and curry powders (it stains and has been used as a dye – Buddhist monks would dye their robes with it). It has a slight earthy, acerbic taste, but for me, the taste is a by-product of a powerful spice.

Anecdotally, its antiseptic properties meant that I went to school numerous times with a bright yellow knee or arm where turmeric had been rubbed onto a graze or a cut by my mother! In Indian weddings turmeric is used in a ceremony the day before the wedding, mixed with flour and made into a dough, which is then rubbed over the bride and bridegroom's skin to lighten, beautify, cleanse and keep them healthy.

Cinnamon

Cinnamon packs one of the highest punches in terms of antioxidants and is number seven in my top ten spices. Antioxidants are necessary to fight the free radicals in our bodies, which can mutate to cause diseases. In short, they keep us healthy. Recently, cinnamon has been heralded as a 'super-spice', as some research has shown that cinnamon can help lower blood sugar levels. It has a light sweet taste so works well in both sweet and savoury dishes, but its winning attribute is that, although it tastes sweet, it doesn't cause blood sugar levels to spike but keeps them stable. This is important to keep digestion calm but also hunger at bay, so a little cinnamon sprinkled on your breakfast is a good way of keeping you away from craving sweet foods during the day.

Cinnamon is native to Sri Lanka but is now grown in India, Brazil, Caribbean and some other parts of the world. It comes from the inner bark and is sold and used whole in a 'quill' shape or ground into a powder. Cinnamon has been embraced as a spice with health properties for many centuries, dating back to the Egyptians who used it for medicinal purposes, embalming bodies, preserving foods and cooking. In Chinese medicine, it is thought to warm the body and help against colds and flu. It smells good and for us evokes cosy scenes of Christmas (candles and soaps are full of this spice at this time of the year), but it is used all year round all over the world. Cinnamon was certainly prized by the Arab spice traders as it commanded a high price due to the long distance traders had to carry it.

Cassia bark (*dalchini*)

This is a type of cinnamon but not from Sri Lanka. It often comes from China and is cheaper to grow than cinnamon. It is darker and 'barkier' in look and a bit harder and less sweet and fragrant than cinnamon. It is used in Indian medicines to calm the stomach and to alleviate feelings of nausea. Indians tend to use cassia bark in both sweet (in rice dishes) and savoury curries and daals. It is also used widely in Chinese cooking and in desserts.

Chillies and chilli powder/chilli flakes

Packed with vitamin C, chillies have seven times the vitamin C level of an orange. Vitamin C is great for keeping colds and illnesses at bay, is an immune booster and is great for overall health. Chillies contain particularly high levels of the antioxidants, vitamin A, many B vitamins, and a wide range of minerals including iron, potassium and manganese. However, it is the active ingredient in chillies, that is causing a stir in diet research. The ingredient that gives chillies, the intense flavour and heat is capsaicin (see p.170), and some research has shown that this helps curb appetite, and the 'heat' this generates can lead to weight loss. Foods that create heat are known as having thermogenic properties and cause us to expend more energy during eating them and for a few hours after too, so this can help for weight loss. Chillies are therefore potential metabolism boosters.

Chillies originate from Mexico and not India as once thought. However, they are prolific and are grown all over the world, with now over 400 varieties.

Cumin seeds

It is thought that cumin originated in the Middle East around Egypt and so is very familiar in Middle Eastern history. It is also grown in India and China. Cumin is featured in ancient history and even referred to in the Old Testament and in Roman and early Greek historical records. It has been found in archaeological sites in Egypt and Syria and was so highly prized that it was used as a currency.

Cumin is an excellent source of iron, a very good source of manganese, and a good source of calcium and magnesium. Iron helps to make red blood cells and these carry oxygen to all the parts of the body. In Ayurvedic medicine and traditionally in India, cumin seeds and powders are used to calm the digestion – the powder is dissolved in hot water and drunk or the seeds are boiled and steeped in hot water to make a warm, soothing tea. Cumin was also used by the Romans instead of black pepper as it has a slight peppery taste. It was also mixed into cosmetics to make the skin look pale. There are also stories of cumin being used as an antiseptic on wounds.

Cumin seeds form the foundation of dishes and spice mixes from around the world – chilli con carne and moles in Mexico, garam masala in India, in Egyptian dukkah and many North African and Moroccan dishes. The seeds are punchy and add pizzazz, fragrance and flavourful warmth to any dish. Roasted and ground, cumin is so fragrant and earthy, it is delicious in salads and is a lovely addition to an average dish, for example, roast beetroot sprinkled with roast cumin is magnificent!

Coriander seeds

Coriander seeds are high in antioxidants, rich in vitamin C and have a high concentration of minerals like potassium, zinc and magnesium, which are vital nutrients for our bodies to function well. Also, coriander seeds in hot water and honey help to soothe menstrual pain and bloating.

In the last few years, we have become very familiar with fresh coriander, which is lovely, green and aromatic. In fact, it is one of the most used culinary herbs. Coriander originated around the Mediterranean and the Middle East. Coriander seeds themselves have been used in foods and medicines for centuries, featuring in Indian, Chinese, Egyptian and Greek history. There is a mention of these seeds in the Old Testament and there is reference in Egyptian and Roman records, endowing coriander seeds with aphrodisiac properties.

Coriander seeds can be used whole, crushed or used fresh as a herb. Coriander seeds when crushed have a slight sweet and citrusy flavour, and when roasted the seeds release a stronger, warmer flavour and aroma. Ground coriander seed adds a wonderful warm depth and taste to dishes, and toasting seeds then grinding them is a good way of getting the full flavour from them.

Cloves

As well as being high in antioxidants, cloves contain vitamins A and C, and the minerals potassium and iron. In Ayurvedic medicine, cloves are believed to contain anti-fungal and anti-inflammatory properties. The strong sweet smell of cloves has led them to be used in breath-freshening products.

This is a spice that is familiar to Europeans as well as Asians, but cloves originally came from the remote Indonesian islands called the Moluccas, but are now cultivated in parts of Africa, India, Pakistan and the West Indies. They were a big part of the spice trade. Cloves are picked as buds from the clove tree. The name 'clove' comes from the French 'clou' which means nail. Clove oil has been used to treat toothache as it has a numbing and antiseptic effect, and in India it is used in drinks and teas to calm the digestion.

Cloves are used in cooking around the world as a spice and in pickles. Chinese five-spice powder, garam masala, roasted Christmas hams, mince pies, and even Worcestershire sauce all contain cloves.

Cardamom

Cardamom is a source of iron and manganese, both nutrients essential to well-being. In Ayuervedic medicine, it is used to soothe digestive problems and to ease nausea and stomach cramps.

There are two types of cardamom. The small green pod is green cardamom, which is familiar to most people, while black cardamom is a larger, black hairy pod. Cardamom is native to India and grows on a bush and the plant is related to the ginger family. It is part of Indian chai, which is a tea made of spices to promote health and with calming properties (it is normally made with cloves, cardamom, cinnamon and fennel seeds). I think of the green cardamom as a festive spice as we often add it to biryanis, sweet rice dishes, and kulfi (ice creams), which are served at celebrations and festivals. It is also used in spice mixes like garam masala. It can be used whole but needs to be slightly opened to release the flavours and aroma. The small, dark seeds inside are very aromatic and are usually used ground into a powder. Cardamom partners well with chocolate, but it is used to flavour both sweet and savoury foods. It is often eaten at the end of a meal in India as it is thought of as a digestive and as a breath freshener.

Black cardamon is used a lot in India and the Far East in curries. It is not as aromatic as the green pod but has a lovely aroma. Black cardamom is also thought to be good for digestion.

Fennel seeds

Fennel seeds are a good source of potassium, magnesium, calcium and vitamins B and C. They have a mild, distinctive aniseed flavour and have been used in the West and the East as a calmative for the stomach and for digestive upsets. Fennel tea is used partly for this and partly as a refreshing drink. Fennel seeds are often eaten in India at the end of a meal to freshen the breath. I suggest drinking hot water infused with fennel seeds during the day, as I believe that this is not only healthy, but keeps the digestion calm and working well.

Grown in parts of the Mediterranean and Asia, fennel seeds are well known and used in both European and Eastern cooking. Many Mediterranean dishes (especially with fish, breads and meats) are cooked with fennel seeds. They are one of the five spices in Chinese five-spice powder and the Bengali panchphoran spice mix.

Carom seeds (also known as bishop's weed)

This spice is not so well known in the West but is one of my favourite seeds. It is closely related to cumin and caraway but has a stronger taste. Carom seeds contain an essential oil called thymol, which is an antiseptic and has anti-inflammatory properties. To me, carom seeds taste like a strong fennel seed but with bite. Its distinctive taste adds a strong warmth to soups, daals, breads, fish and meats. In my family and all over India, it is the go-to and routine spice to alleviate stomach pain and indigestion. Chewing a small handful (they do taste bitter) is an everyday remedy to stop nausea, indigestion, ease stomach upsets and helps with bloating too. Steeping a few seeds in hot water and drinking as a tea is also thought to work as a remedy for asthma.

Fenugreek seeds

Fenugreek seeds contain lots of vitamins, minerals and are rich in antioxidants. In India, we use them to relieve arthritic pain and they are thought to be very good for the digestion.

Native to the Mediterranean and India, they are small, light brown-orange seeds found in a pod, and are used in Greek, Mediterranean and Asian cuisine. Originally, the plant was grown by the Greeks as cattle fodder. This spice comes to life when roasted or cooked as it releases a strong pungent smell but a taste that can transform a whole dish with a unique delicious flavour. Fresh fenugreek leaves are small but highly aromatic. They are wonderful in salads, breads, curries and bhajis. The dried leaves are perfect added to the end of a dish to lift the flavour (you only need a small amount). The dried seeds are ideal for releasing a pungent oil when cooking soups and pickles. Fenugreek seeds are also used in curry powder mixes.

Sumac

Prepare yourself for a bit of stardust!
Sumac is cultivated in the Middle East and around the Mediterranean. It comes from the berries of a

plant that are dried and then ground. Sumac is a tangy, lemony spice, which is used throughout the Mediterranean, African subcontinent, Middle East and in Persian dishes. It is not only beautiful (a deep red brick colour) but a zingy, taste-boosting spice that adds magic to so many dishes. Sumac is full of vitamin C and antioxidants and can elevate the taste in dishes – try adding a sprinkling to roast sweet potatoes or on your favourite hummus dish or rub into a roast chicken.

Za'atar
This is a spectacular mix of herbs, thyme, sesame seeds, sumac and sometimes cumin, and is a staple of Middle East cooking. The ingredients can vary slightly sometimes and may include dried marjoram. All these ingredients, however, have good health benefits. Thyme is a lovely herb full of antioxidants, and sesame seeds are rich in iron, calcium and vitamin B.

Ras el hanout
This literally means 'the top of the shop', i.e. the best in the spice shop! It is a heady mix of anything between 12 and 100 spices including dried peppers, cardamom, nutmeg, allspice, cinnamon, cloves, fennel, ginger, turmeric, rose buds and lavender.

Saffron
This is the most expensive spice in the world. It has been used in the East and West for centuries, in everything from risottos to tagines to curries and delicious desserts.

Saffron is native to Persia. It comes from the dried stigmas from the flowers of the saffron crocus. It is expensive as it has to be hand picked and it takes thousands of stigmas to generate a tiny amount of saffron. It has been linked to helping against depression and contains vitamins, minerals and a mammoth amount of manganese, which helps to control blood sugar levels. It also has an amazing flavour – almost bitter, but also sweet. It transcends dishes with its flavour and it adds a beautiful golden colour to dishes. Saffron is best used by infusing it in water or milk, or roasting and then adding to dishes. A small amount goes a long way.

Szechuan pepper
This is a fantastic spice and has a unique, distinctive taste. Spicy, lemony, tingly on your tongue and slightly fizzy, but don't let this put you off. Szechuan pepper comes from the berries of a prickly ash tree. When ripe, the berries split open to reveal the seeds, but it is the beautiful pink husk that holds the fragrant, almost addictive flavour. Szechuan peppers are different to traditional black peppercorns. They have been used in traditional Chinese medicines for centuries and are one of the staple ingredients in Chinese five-spice powder. They release their aroma when roasted or cooked and are best eaten ground (they may need sieving as the husk is hard to grind into a fine powder) or used to flavour hot oil and then removed before eating. As their taste feels numbing, they have been used in Chinese medicine to treat toothache. They are also used to treat digestion problems. Szechuan peppers contain a host of vitamins including vitamins A and K, and minerals, such as potassium, zinc and selenium.

The import of Szechuan pepper was banned in the USA for years by the Department of Agriculture as it was thought to carry a bacterium that could kill citrus crops. This ban was lifted in 2005 to the relief of many people who had missed the lovely taste of this distinctive spice.

Star anise
Star anise is the fruit of an evergreen plant native to China. One of the most beautiful-looking spices, this dark brown star-shaped spice has an exotic shape and a deep liquorice flavour. It is used mainly in Chinese and Vietnamese cuisine and is used to add a depth of flavour to dishes, including the Vietnamese Pho broth. Star anise is also one of the ingredients in Chinese five-spice powder. We also use it in India, particularly in rice dishes, and it also adds a lovely sweet flavour to fruit-based desserts. In Chinese medicine, it is thought to have many health properties including as an anti-spasmodic to ease digestion. Star anise contains shikimic acid, which is thought to prevent flu. For a small spice, it is a great source of vitamins A, B and C.

Spicy DOESN'T Always Mean Hot!

So often when you say 'spicy', it immediately conjures up mouth-burning, sweat-inducing food. How wrong can you be?

The word 'spice' refers to plants, seeds and fruits. It doesn't mean just chillies or hot spices. In fact, most spices add aroma, a diverse or singular flavour and sometimes a sweetness, depending on the actual spice. Spices such as cinnamon add a natural sweetness, cloves add a gentle tingle, and Szechuan peppers are citrusy rather than 'chilli' hot. Cardamom, fennel and fenugreek are beautifully aromatic, star anise has a liquorice sweet taste, and turmeric has a slightly earthy, bitter taste. Spices also have wonderful effects on your senses – Szechuan peppers make the tongue tingle happily, while fennel seeds and green cardamom seeds leave a fresh sweet breath in your mouth.

In the Middle East and Iran, spices are used for their intense flavour and aroma rather than for heat. For example, sumac adds a distinct lemony taste to dishes, or saffron is used as colouring as well as for its individual semi-sweet and almost bitter flavour.

Heat can come from some spices and peppers, but the most common understanding of 'heat' is from certain chillies. There are over 400 varieties of chillies in the world and not all chillies are hot. It's a real shame that chillies have acquired a bad name as some add a mild, smoky flavour, like chipotle chillies, which is a smoked dried jalapeño chilli. Going to Indian restaurants and ordering the hottest dish as a dare has become synonymous with eating chillies, but many chillies just give a small, welcome kick to dishes, adding a unique dimension to them. In fact, many people across the world who use chilli in their food prefer the mild or medium varieties and stay away from chillies that blow your head off! The old picture of Indian cooking being either a sweet korma at one end or a fiery vindaloo at the other is a myth! Most Indian cooking is so varied. It is milder and creamier in the north and has a lovely multilayered hot, coconut, creamy and sour flavour in the south, with many taste variations geographically and culturally in between.

How to spot a hot chilli

Trying to spot a hot chilli is quite difficult. Heat is an individual thing – some people can take very hot spice and some can't tolerate even a little. However, it is good to know the variety of the chilli before using it. I do try them raw first, but I wouldn't encourage you to do this.

If you don't know the variety, you can tone down the heat by removing the seeds and membrane from the chilli. The heat comes from the membranes that are attached to the seeds. Do this carefully with gloves or wash your hands straight away! You don't want to rub your eyes (or other parts) with chilli hands as this can sting and hurt. If you do eat a hot chilli and your mouth is burning, the antidote is not something sweet, but cold milk or yogurt. This is because the heat comes from capsaicin, the active compound contained in the chillies which triggers a burning sensation when we eat it. Drinking milk will help to neutralise this effect as the protein in the dairy helps to break down the heat from the capsaicin compound.

There is a measure of hotness in chillies called the Scoville scale. This scale ranges from 0 for bell peppers to 2,200 for the Carolina reaper! Chilli names such as scorpion, naga (meaning snake), viper and ghost pepper should give you a big hint that these aren't chillies to be trifled with! I have to say that I'm not sure if I would ever try these or think of cooking with them. I have listed here some that are more readily available and also some of the ones that I have used for the recipes in this book in terms of their 'hotness'. This is my list, but please be aware that this is my own personal interpretation.

Starting from the very hot end:

- Habanero and Scotch bonnet – Used in Caribbean and some South American regions. You will find these in some very hot Caribbean sauces.
- Bird's eye chillies – These are from the Far East and are small, red and fiery. I use these when I want a very hot hit! Normally used in Thai and Vietnamese curries, they are very hot, so handle carefully and use them in small amounts.
- Piri piri – These can vary in heat but are genarally quite hot and are found in Portugal, Brazil and some parts of Africa.
- Cayenne chilli – This is from Cayenne and we would normally see it as a dried powder or often used in dried chilli flakes.
- Serrano pepper – A chilli from Mexico with a medium heat.
- Aleppo peppers – These chillies are from the Syrian town of Aleppo and are mild and have a smoky flavour and lovely red, rusty colour.
- Jalapeño chilli – Mexican quite mild chilli.
- Chipotle – A smoke-dried jalapeño chilli which is mild and smoky in flavour, it is used in Mexican and TexMex dishes.
- Ancho – This is a dried poblano pepper. It is mild and is used in Mexican mole sauces and gives a rich, deep flavour.
- Padrón – These are small Spanish peppers. They are mainly mild but every now and then a hot one creeps in. They are delicious cooked simply in a little olive oil and salt as a tapas dish.
- Paprika – Made from a mild red pepper, which is air-dried, Spanish paprika is often smoked. It is used all over the Middle East and probably came to our notice through dishes such as Hungarian goulash and Spanish paella.
- Kashmiri chillies – These are used in Indian cooking and are mild. They add a lovely, natural red colour to dishes. I love using these in my spice rubs.

In this book most of the recipes that refer to red chillies are mild to medium chillies (usually long) found in supermarkets. Green chillies are the variety from India and Kenya, which are more medium to hot. Thai bird's eye chillies are very hot.

Chilli powders
I often buy red whole dried chillies and grind them into a powder or flakes. This means that I know exactly what is in my powder – sometimes powdered chillies may have colours added to them or a mix of chillies.

Chilli flakes
Sometimes the chilli flakes in shop-bought jars have little potency and the flakes are rather large, so when you cook with them, the result is bland and the flakes get stuck in your teeth! Buy whole dried red chillies and grind these to the size of flakes that you like, then store in an airtight container.

Index

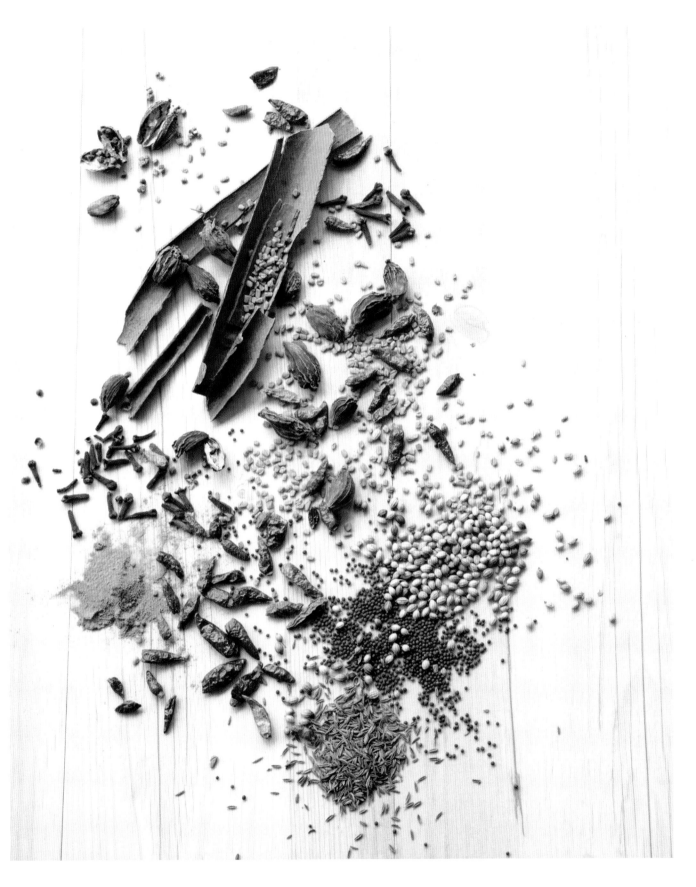

Acknowledgements

I have been secretly nurturing the idea for this book for years. Eventually I nervously shared it with cookery book writer, Jenny Chandler, and she was so lovely and encouraging, putting me in touch with the illustrious Emily Preece-Morrison at Pavilion. Emily's reaction to the idea and her enthusiasm, unwavering belief, determination and gentle guidance has brought this idea to fruition.

Emily handpicked the most calm, wonderful team who brought their immense creative skills to this book – chic and funny prop stylist Wei Tang, infinitely stylish food stylist Rosie Reynolds, lovely designer Laura Russell and THE very best photographer, Claire Winfield. Anita Bean, who worked out the calorie counts, and copy editor Kathy Steer were also invaluable.

There are people in life who make a real difference and I have 'Energised Kim' (Kim Ingleby), who has been my mentor and coach for years, who was as excited as I was about my book from the very beginning and had so much faith in me. I think the turning point for me in my confidence was winning the Asian Women's Achievement Award in 2013 and meeting one of the most brilliant Asian women, Pinky Lilani. Pinky has inspired me as a role model in being not only successful, but also understanding the moral responsibility which comes with that.

There are two other people who gave me the conviction to write this book. When I asked her the question 'does this idea have legs?' food writer extraordinaire Xanthe Clay immediately said 'oh yes!' and I have been privileged to have her support. It takes real belief to help someone through a project from beginning to end and Sam Goldsmith (recipe consultant and friend) helped me, not only by testing so many of my recipes, but by teaching me so much about recipe writing and putting together a food book. Bringing his schoolteacher discipline to my writing kept me on track!

I consider myself so lucky to have had so much support and encouragement from so many friends and family – my wonderful son, Benjamin, who loves to eat and makes me so happy when he does, my husband Mark, with his never-ending support and love for me and my lovely family (my mum, my amazing sisters, Sandhya, Savita and Kavita and my brother, Ravi) who I know are always proud of everything I do and Audrey, Howard, Nicole, Karen, Simon, Sophie and Nick. A special thanks too to Alan W.

Thank you to so many of my friends who have tested my recipes: Darpan, Sophie, Jon and Jenny. Barbara, Pete, Hannah, Jane and Kate and thanks also to Ed Boal of Gregg Latchams, Sachin for my website and Natasha for helping me when I was shaking sending the final text to Emily! Finally, I have included in the book a tribute recipe to my eldest sister, Mohinder, who passed away some years ago and who was by far and away the best cook in the family and who loved cooking for us.

First published in paperback in the United Kingdom in 2019 by Pavilion
43 Great Ormond Street
London
WC1N 3HZ

Text © Kalpna Woolf, 2015, 2019
Photography, design and layout © Pavilion Books Company Ltd, 2015, 2019

Photographer: Clare Winfield

ISBN: 978-1-911641-30-8

A CIP catalogue record for this book is available from the British Library.

10 9 8 7 6 5 4 3 2 1

Reproduction by Colour Depth, UK
Printed and bound by 1010 Printing International Ltd, China

www.pavilionbooks.com

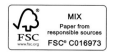